BODYWISE

BODY

Regaining
natural flexibility
for maximum

JOSEPH HELLER &

JEREMY P. TARCHER, INC.
Los Angeles

WISE

your
and vitality
well-being

WILLIAM A. HENKIN

Distributed by St. Martin's Press
New York

Library of Congress Cataloging in Publication Data

Heller, Joseph, 1940–
Bodywise.

 Bibliography: p. 245
 Includes index.
 1. Health. 2. Mind and body. 3. Body, Human.
I. Henkin, William, 1944–   . II. Title.
RA776.H485 1986 613 86-3757
ISBN 0-87477-391-1
ISBN 0-87477-386-5 (pbk.)

Jeremy P. Tarcher, Inc.
9110 Sunset Blvd.
Los Angeles, CA 90069

Design by Kitty Maryatt, Two Hands Press
Illustration by Rex Norman, Jackie Entwistle, and Valerie Deo

Manufactured in the United States of America
10 9 8 7 6 5 4 3 2 1

First Edition

The authors wish to thank the following for permission to reprint
material:

Robert M. Martin for photographic material from *The Gravity
Guiding System*. Gravity Guidance, Inc., 1982, Pasadena.

Even Cowgirls Get the Blues by Tom Robbins. Copyright © 1976
by Thomas Robbins. Reprinted by permission of Bantam Books,
Inc. All rights reserved.

Harcourt-Brace for material from *The Lovesong of J. Alfred
Prufrock* by T. S. Eliot © 1930, 1934.

The Prophet by Kahlil Gibran, by permission of Alfred A. Knopf,
Inc. Copyright © 1923 by Kahlil Gibran and renewed 1951 by
Administrators C.T.A. of Kahlil Gibran Estate, and Mary G. Gibran.

Jim Russi for photographic material from *Surfer Magazine*.
Copyright © 1986, *Surfer Magazine*.

CONTENTS

Also by William A. Henkin

The Psychic Healing Book, coauthored with Amy
Wallace

ACKNOWLEDGMENTS

For their contributions to our bodies and knowledge, the authors wish to thank

Cindy Stone Butler, Joanne Sutro Cain, Andy Crow, Vern Haddick, Catherine Keir, Sylvia Randall, Sophia Reinders, Ida Rolf, Peter Rutter, Don St. John, Kensho David Schneider, Stephanie Willet-Shaw.

PART ONE: KNOWLEDGE OF BODY

THE BODY IN EVERYDAY LIFE

1

THE NATURE OF THE BEAST

As you read these words, what is your body doing? How are you holding your hands and arms? Your feet? Your back? Your head? What sorts of sensations are you having in your muscles, bones, and nerves? Do you feel light? Tense? Relaxed? Rigid? When did you last check in with yourself this way?

It would be hard to get along in this life without a body, and yet, to some extent, this is exactly what most of us try to do. We trust our physical forms to do their animal-like jobs of moving us through the world, while we—whoever or whatever we may think "we" are—proceed with the rational, emotional, and spiritual work of judging and evaluating our feelings and behaviors, codifying our thoughts and experiences, and contemplating our navels.

As long as our bodies do what we imagine they are supposed to do, we pay them little attention. Some food here, a bath there, and an occasional workout of the large muscle groups or the cardiovascular system to help us maintain the illusion that we are not moving inexorably toward death—these activities comprise most of the concern we exhibit for the intricate packages we seem to inhabit for the few short decades of our residence on Earth. For most of us, a "body" is something an "I" owns, like a car or a dog. Except when something goes wrong with the mechanism and we experience illness or disease, or when we "lose ourselves" in the rare transports of physical ecstasy that can result from an exceptional sensual experience, we rarely even attempt to understand the relationship between our bodies and our "selves."

To some degree the very structure of our language has established, encouraged, and reinforced this conceptual separation between our bodies and the rest of us. To say, for example, "I have a headache," is to make it sound as if you have taken possession of this thing, this ache, that was outside and separate from yourself. It is as if out there in the universe some headache was floating around that no one owned, and you grabbed it, went out and acquired it for your head, and now it is yours. Or perhaps you went running this morning, and when you came home you said, "My legs are tired," as if your legs are somehow separate and different from your body or from you. In our language it would sound peculiar to say "I ache in my head," or "I am tired in my legs." And even though these sentences are more accurate than the ones we commonly use, they still create artificial separations exactly like the distinctions between the body and the "I."

If this sounds like a lot of fuss about a little point, consider how small a step it is between separating your head from your body and separating your body from you. These ideas may make various sorts of conceptual sense, but they pose insurmountable functional problems, since at least in this life your body and head could no more get along without each other than could your body and your self.

This notion, borrowed from general semantics theory, is explored more fully in such books as Alfred Korzybski's *Science and Sanity* and Benjamin Whorf's *Language, Thought, and Reality.* The central thesis is that the way in which we construct our language shapes our perception of reality. The structure of a sentence itself dictates a relationship between the parts of that sentence. We then project that relationship into the relationship whose reality we have attempted to describe with the sentence in the first place.

In languages more primitive than ours, reality is described differently. For instance, we have abstracted a concept called "legs" that we apply indiscriminately to people, tables, animals, triangles, ideas—"He doesn't have a leg to stand on"—and so forth. A so-called primitive culture may not abstract that concept; instead, it may have one word for a horse's legs, another for human legs, and no leglike word at all for the branches of a triangle. The classic example of this difference among languages and cultural perceptions is that people who live in tropical and temperate climates have very few ways to distinguish among different kinds of snow, whereas some Eskimo tribes have two dozen words, each of which qualitatively specifies a particular variation of snow. The Eskimos have accomplished something with their language that is beyond our perceptual and linguistic capabilities. On the other hand, we have accomplished the task, beyond *their* capabilities, of abstracting, out of twenty-eight different things they see, a single common entity called snow.

As if in reaction to this divorce of body from soul, a few modern students of the body have redefined the identity of the first person singular. At a bioenergetics

What is first to be considered is that the organism always works as a whole. We *have* not a liver or a heart. We *are* liver and heart and brain and so on, and even this is wrong. We are not a summation of parts, but a *coordination*—a very subtle coordination of all these different bits that go into the making of the organism.
—Fritz Perls, *Gestalt Therapy Verbatim*

Holography is a method of lensless photography in which the wave field of light scattered by an object is recorded on a plate as an interference pattern. When the photographic record—the hologram—is placed in a coherent light beam like a laser, the original wave pattern is regenerated. A three-dimensional image appears.

Because there is no focusing lens, the plate appears as a meaningless pattern of swirls. *Any piece of the hologram will reconstruct the entire image.* [3]

workshop, for instance, Ken Dychtwald "stopped 'having' a body and first began to realize that I 'am' my body and that my body 'is' *me.* "[1] Similarly, Stanley Keleman "felt that I did not inhabit my body, I *was* my body."[2] In the pages that follow we neither assume that we *own* our bodies nor that we *are* them. Rather, we regard the body as an aspect of a puzzle that, when combined with other aspects commonly called the mind and spirit, forms the integrated unit of a whole person.

THE BODY AS THE HOLOGRAM OF THE BEING

The body is the hologram of the being. In an abstract sense it may be seen as an exact physical expression of a person's mind and spirit, manifesting the thoughts, emotions, intuitions, and everything else that make a person both unique and distinctly human. In a concrete sense, any part of the body may be seen to reflect and contain everything there is to know about the whole body, just as any part of a holographic image will reproduce the entire image, albeit with reduced intensity and less specific data.

If you cut off the ear from a hologram of an entire face and place the image of the ear in a laser beam, you will not end up with a picture of an ear, but with a picture of a little ear-sized face. Just as the piece of a hologram reflects the entire holographic image, so any part of the body reflects the condition of the entire being—physical, mental, emotional, and spiritual. This is why a well-trained bodyworker can read a great deal about a person's psyche and history just by studying the body.

The holographic approach underlies two basic themes in this book: First, that one can read, approach, or interact with the whole human being in all his parts and manifestations through the body; and second, that considering the whole body, rather than one or some of its parts, provides readier access to more of a person's dimensions than dealing with any one of its aspects.

The body is not only the hologram of the being, it is also home. However we understand the mind-body separation most of us take for granted, it is immediately apparent that as human beings we could not have our mental, emotional, or spiritual lives if we did not have our bodies. No great scientists have had their intellectual insights, no great lovers have felt their deep passions, no spiritual masters have experienced higher consciousness, without their bodies. In all these instances, only the focus of the person's attention has moved outside his or her body. But there is no way to have any kind of out-of-body experience without a body to have it out of.

When body and mind function as an integral unit—what Ken Dychtwald refers to as "bodymind," and what might even more appropriately, if more awkwardly, be called "bodymindspirit"—the energy of life flows freely. When the components are perceived separately, the energy of life becomes dammed up and stagnant, just as pools cut off from flowing rivers get gummy with muck and debris. In the human being those stagnant pools manifest both psychologically and somatically as pain, tension, rigidity, and malfunction. This is how a stuck body holographically reflects a stuck being, and a free body reflects a free being.

Another useful way to understand the body is as a biofeedback mechanism for the here and now. Compare it with, say, a Geiger counter, which is useful only as long as it keeps reading the radiation in its environment at the moment it is operating. If for some reason the Geiger counter has a memory, and reflects a reading of some past session while it is supposed to be reflecting the present, the information it provides misleads the reader.

This is exactly the problem we have as human beings. Our memories are valuable when we can exercise

Our holographic perception of the body is partly derived from general systems theory, enunciated in 1937 by Ludwig von Bertalanffy, which states that a change in any component of an integrated system will alter the entire system.

For our purposes, general systems theory implies that "if one part of the body is ill, the functioning of other aspects is affected. A headache [for example] will decrease one's appetite and one's desire for body movement, socialization, or study."[4] While we cannot completely control the systems that are the body and the being just by understanding them, understanding what happens to our feet when something changes in our shoulders may allow us to begin to move *toward* such control.

them at will. But when we are unaware of the difference between a reading of the past and one of the present, or when we are unaware that the past is what we are interpreting in the present, we can only grow confused.

It is well established that physical as well as psychological problems may result from unresolved experiences in our past. Our bodies always live in the here and now, but our awareness often lags behind, playing and replaying different variations of past events. The events from your past are now inscribed upon the tablet of your flesh, and today your body shows your life story so clearly that anyone who has learned to read the body can tell the approximate nature and time of your major physical and emotional traumas without asking you a single question. You already have a past, which dominates your life to some degree. This book is going to give you a present.

WHAT THIS BOOK CAN DO FOR YOU

The purpose of this book is to explain something of the way all human bodies function in order to give you a greater ability to feel alive in your own body; to have more pleasure and fewer problems with it; and to explore its interconnections with other parts of the universe, beginning with your own multifaceted self. Whether you are a physician, a physiotherapist, a bodyworker, a nurse, an athlete, a dancer, a person suffering from muscular or skeletal pain, tension, stress, and discomfort, or simply someone who wants to live easily and gracefully in the physical world, you will find that the body's inherent flexibility fairly begs you to live a life of ease, balance, and integrity—and that doing so is possible.

This book will show you a way to perceive and think about your body that will enable you to move more efficiently and gracefully than you do at present, and to live a physical life whose greater ease and balance can reduce pain, stress, tension, and discomfort. It explains some things you can and cannot do to improve your physical functioning by arriving at a new way to understand and think about your body, and by living the principles of that understanding. In this way, it can be a tool that will help you to perceive whether, where, and why some sort of bodywork might be beneficial to you.

In the first part of this book, "Knowledge of Body," we examine some of the ideas that underlie all kinds of bodywork, and one kind—the structural integration called Hellerwork—in particular. In the first three chapters, we examine some of the ways in which your body and mind are connected, and some of the ways in which your body's systems work together as *biofunctional* units —interconnected groups of muscles, bones, and organs —rather than as anatomical units; then, in Chapter 4, we discuss the system of Hellerwork itself. In Part Two, "Body of Knowledge," we explore your body according to its biofunctional systems, with easy exercises that will move you along on your path to a life of increasing grace and flexibility. In the course of the book we invite you repeatedly to learn about your body through physical experiences. The exercises and experiments you find here and there in our text are all designed to help you incorporate some of what we discuss, so that you can actually learn about the body *from* the body—your body —while you are reading this book.

This is not exactly a do-it-yourself book, however. Books full of techniques and exercises designed to make you better already exist, and if you have read them and tried to follow their instructions, you know that in the long run they do not work. Why? Because they assume that fundamental changes can be effected in your body simply by changing what you do with it. This is inaccurate. You cannot alter physical *functioning* in any meaningful way without altering physical *structure* first, and written prescriptions by themselves cannot lead you to alter physical structure much; hands-on bodywork can accomplish this sort of change most effectively.

What words *can* do, and what this book does, is give you a sense of your own possibilities and provide guidance so that you can achieve them. For example, if you run with your feet turned out and your weight falling back on your heels, no book in the world will improve the problems you have with turnout, which reflect the habits of your physical structure. But this book will explain your physical structure to you so that you can start to move with better balance, with your weight more evenly distributed over your whole foot. Then, when you feel the ways in which your body's structure determines the degree of stress you feel, you can make a meaningful choice about the kinds of exercise or bodywork you want in order to bring your feet into line and to feel best in and about your body.

We make no assumption in the following pages that the body is "better" or "more" than the mind, spirit, or personality. The whole of a person is greater than the sum of his or her parts, and the nature of a person's integrity can be perceived most easily through the hologram that is the human body.

THE BODY AS PATTERN INTEGRITY

"Few of us have lost our minds," Ken Wilber writes, "but most of us have long ago lost our bodies."[5] Wilber does not mean that we have lost our physical bodies, of course, but rather that we have lost an *awareness* of our bodies as real parts of our real selves. We have come to regard them as suspiciously alien *things,* and while they may provide us with pleasure on occasion, we know they are bound to betray us in the end. Looking at our bodies in this way, we fail to grasp their importance as providers of information and executors of our wills.

The body is not a "deeper reality" than the ego, as some somatologists think, but the *integration* of the body *and* the ego is indeed a deeper reality than either alone. . . .
—Ken Wilber, *No Boundary*

Integrity: 1. The condition of having no part or element taken away or wanting; undivided or unbroken state; material wholeness, completeness, entirety.
—*Oxford English Dictionary*

In the realm of the soma, things are what they seem and energies can be measured quantitatively in terms of the movements they produce.
—Alexander Lowen, *The Language of the Body*

10

Even though the body is the solid aspect of our existence, it is always in the process of change. Blood is flowing, cells are dying and rebuilding, chemical structure is altering—nothing really remains static. Every cell in your body is replaced every seven years; yet, while your flesh is completely different, it is still quite identifiably *your body*. The sameness/differentness reflects the Buddhist notion of reincarnation, which Walpola Rahula describes as a candle burning. The flame when a candle is first lit and the flame when the candle is nearly gone are clearly not the same flame; yet just as clearly they are not different flames. Instead, the fire that burns throughout the life of the candle is "a series that continues unbroken, but changes every moment. That series is . . . nothing but movement . . ."[6]

Buckminster Fuller called this kind of serial process *pattern integrity.* He illustrated pattern integrity by supposing that you take a cotton rope and tie it to the end of a silk rope, and tie the silk rope to the end of a sisal rope, and then make a knot in the top of the cotton rope. As you slide the knot down through the cotton rope, through the silk rope, through the sisal rope, it is first a cotton knot, then a silk knot, then a sisal knot. Each time it moves from one rope to the next, nothing is the same about it except the integral pattern we call the knot. Like Rahula's flame, and like Fuller's knot, your body *is* a process of change, of movement, whose integrity is inherent in its pattern.

The process of change our bodies are in is reflected both in our understandings of our bodies and of the experiences we encounter through them. Wherever you are right now, reach out with your hand and touch some hard object—a stone, a wall, a piece of metal or wood—and feel its hardness. Now, stroke that same object with the same hand, and feel its texture and temperature. Rough or smooth, warm or cool, it is the same object that was hard a moment ago. It is not less hard now, but the information it gives you is different because you transformed your experience of the object through the conscious use of your body.

Of course, you do not experience the hard object with your body alone; you experience it with your whole self. Each aspect of yourself—mental, physical, emotional, spiritual—works with all the others, sharing information for the benefit of the integrated person that you are. You may find it delightful to eat a fine meal or to make love, but if you were only a mind you would find it difficult to have such experiences. At the same time, if you were only a body, who could interpret the physical experience and let you know you're having a good time? The human response to the world is neither physiological nor psychological. It is psychophysiological.

THE BODY DISOWNED

Since at least the time when Plato organized the human being's components into a hierarchy, with reason and the mind standing above the desires and motivations of the spirit, and with the appetites of the physical body lurking at the bottom, we in the Western world have tried to disown the body. Sometimes we feel justified for doing so, as when we close off awareness of chronic pain in order to release ourselves from its unpleasant feelings. But when we protect ourselves from experiences we do not like, we simultaneously close ourselves off from the possibility of experiences we might like very much. Just as a thick wall that protects us from a bullet also prevents us from receiving a loving caress, so a body that is insensitive to pain is equally insensitive to pleasure.

Moreover, as we close down our sense of pain, any affliction that causes pain does not go away; it merely disappears from our consciousness. The cause of the pain remains, even though we have ceased to be aware of it, and we devote great energy to protecting ourselves both from the pain and from the knowledge that we are in pain.

To get a sense of how such suppressed pain can sap your energy, make a fist. Squeeze that fist tight. Tighter. Tighter still. Good. Keep squeezing. What other muscles can you feel that tightened up without your meaning them to do so? Release your fist. How much of your hand feels relieved? How much of your arm? The rest of your body? How much mental attention, both conscious and unconscious, was on maintaining the pressure in your fist, arm, and the rest of your body, that is now free for other matters? This is the way pain, tension, stress, and discomfort occupy the energies by which you live. This is the way these sensations make you tired and keep you from expressing yourself in creative, fulfilling ways. The fact that some muscles in your body grew taut without your knowledge, simply to support the flection in your fist, did not stress your arm any less than if you *had* known they were growing tight. In fact, it may have caused considerably *more* stress. Now that you are aware of the relationship between energy and tension (or pain, or stress, or discomfort), make a fist again, and see how few muscles are really needed to do so and how much energy you save.

If you have ever had a severe headache or cramps, you know how fatiguing even a minor pain can be. Most of us are in constant pain in some parts of our bodies already, without even realizing it, and we are directing our creative, expressive, loving, and expansive energies to hiding the pain from our awareness. We are not so much wasting energy when we do this sort of thing as we are spending it unwisely and inefficiently. As coming chapters in this book will show, we could, instead, release our bodies as well as our minds from pain and use our energy for greater pleasure, fulfillment, and satisfaction.

As this book proceeds, we will explore the divorce of body from mind, and we will examine some of the physical and psychological distortions and dis-ease that result from creating an artificial barrier between body and mind. We will also take a look at some of the ways somatologists and bodyworkers have discovered to heal the split, and at some of the benefits that can result from making ourselves whole again.

For the purposes of this book, "dis-ease" does not mean illness, particularly. As Robert S. DeRopp points out, it is "simply a way of saying 'absence of ease' in two syllables."[7] And dis-ease is exactly what we want to eliminate and avoid by learning more about our bodies.

THE BODY'S ROLE IN THE STRUCTURES OF CONSCIOUSNESS

2

THE BODY AND THE WORLD

There is an ancient Chinese story related by Chuang Tzu of a Taoist butcher who had not had his knives sharpened for twenty years; yet they were as finely honed as they had been on the day they were new. When the local king heard of this remarkable phenomenon he had the butcher brought before him and asked how such a miracle was possible. The butcher explained that an ordinary cook has to sharpen his knives every month because he hacks at his meat, while a good cook has only to sharpen his knives every year because he cuts and carves; but he, himself, was in the Way, and wherever his knife blade went the flesh was already parting, and so his blades never wore down.

Many forces affect us all the time. When we are at ease and at peace and in balance with our circumstances we experience those forces as complementary, and our blades can last for years and years. When we are not in harmony with the world around us we experience the forces as antagonistic, and the conflict between them results in friction that tires us out and wears down all our blades.

In the traditions of Western society we tend to seek peace with our surroundings by forcing them to accommodate us, in which case we deem ourselves victorious, or by submitting to them, in which case we think we are defeated. Our perspective derives from perceiving an either/or universe, a place of polar opposites. For instance, we see ourselves in good health until some breakdown occurs, and then we see ourselves as ill. In fact, health is a continuum of body functioning that runs from total well-being at one end to total breakdown at the other. At all times we are moving somewhere along this continuum. When we realize that health is not just a matter of being well or ill, we can perceive a variety of physical states, all of which are more or less healthy.

The practice of preventive medicine is based on the perception that health exists on such a continuum, and that we see ourselves simply as well or ill—*only* at one extreme or the other—as a consequence of living out of balance and therefore in a state of conflict. The friction of resistance, destruction, and wear that results from such an existence presses on us—oppresses us, suppresses us, depresses us—until we are compressed in body, mind, and spirit.

When we perceive opposing forces to be complementary, on the other hand, they combine so that every force contributes to every other force, and no single force is unnecessary to the whole.

The body reflects the conditions of our relationship with the world around us. For example, when you look at your body do you see a figure with bent legs and bowed shoulders, dragging its feet and staring at the ground? Perhaps this body will alert you to a chronic feeling that life is a heavy burden. Do you see a figure with chest thrust forward and shoulders thrown back, stomach tucked in and head held high? Such a body might tell you that you have challenged and defied your life. Or do you see a body whose head is evenly balanced on its neck, whose shoulders, hips, and ankles are aligned, that moves with easy fluidity, and which seems calmly attuned to the circumstances of every moment as it comes? This is a body that tells you it is at home in the world.

Whatever shape your body is in, however, it has supported and served you well so far. You are more alive than dead, you are more out of pain than in it, and you are more in than out of balance—as you know because you don't fall over when you stand up. But no matter what shape your body is in, there is still room for improvement: not just in the quantity of support your body can provide, not necessarily in its ability to support you *more,* but in the quality of that support, in your body's ability to serve you *better.* In this chapter we shall explore some of the ways our bodies affect our perceptions of reality. We shall see how a body that is out of balance perceives a world that is out of balance, how a body that is misaligned experiences the world as misaligned, and how, when we transform our bodies, we may find the world we live in transformed as well. We may find, in other words, that the flesh of life can part before the blade of our physical passage.

THE BODY AS THE UNCONSCIOUS

When we refer to "I" or "me," we generally mean that nebulous sense of self-awareness to which we attribute "consciousness." Are you conscious of yourself at this moment? How do you experience that self? Exactly what about yourself are you conscious *of?* Your feelings? Your mind? Your spirit? Your body?

Here is a simple exercise from Ken Wilber's book, *No Boundary,* that will acquaint you not so much with your body as with the extent to which you are aware of it. Lie down on your back, stretched out on a bed, mat, or rug. Then:

> Simply close your eyes, breathe deeply but easily, and begin to explore your bodily feelings. Don't *try* to feel anything, don't force feelings, just let your attention flow through your body and note if any feeling, positive or negative, is present in the various parts of your body. Can you, for example, feel your legs? Your stomach? Your heart? Eyes? Genitals, buttocks, scalp, diaphragm, feet? Notice which parts of the body feel alive with feeling, full and strong and vital, and which parts seem dull, heavy, lifeless, dimmed, tight, or painful. Try this for at least three minutes, and notice how often your attention might leave the body and wander into daydreams. Does it strike you as odd that it might be very difficult to stay in your body for three minutes? If you're not in your body, where are you?[1]

As you can see from performing this little exercise, we are often detached from all but the most incidental awareness of our bodies. The surprising implication is that we rely on the body's automaticity far more than we might imagine. Despite the fact that we think of ourselves as rational beings, and that rational is even offered by most dictionaries as one definition of sane, it is our nonrational, unconscious aspects that govern most facets of our lives most of the time.

Our unconscious functioning is essential not only for autonomic functions like breathing air, circulating blood, and digesting food; it also protects us in many ways. For instance, when you touch a hot stove you pull your hand away even before you are aware of the stove's heat. If you carefully monitor your behavior and thoughts over the course of a single day—or a single hour, or even, as the exercise above demonstrates, for three minutes—you

The body *is* the unconscious.
—Mary Whitehouse

will find that most of what you think, feel, say, and do happens automatically. This automaticity is the very embodiment of the domination of the unconscious in our lives.

To see the power of another kind of unconscious process, habit, try the following experiment: Cross your arms. Now cross them the other way. Did you have any problem carrying out the second instruction? There is no innate anatomical difference between crossing your arms one way and crossing them another way; there is no "reason" for the difficulty most people have. You have simply learned to use your body according to a pattern that you repeated and repeated until it became *your* way —and you did so without thinking about what you were doing. Crossing your arms one way rather than another is not a dangerous, painful, or debilitating movement pattern, although there are probably others you have taken on that are equally ingrained and that *do* cause you pain or stress. Many unconscious patterns are particularly insidious because they appear so innocuously in our lives —in the ways we sit, stand, walk, and bend over, for example. It is even possible to lie down and sleep in a position that adds to your stress rather than diminishing it.

There is nothing inherently wrong with having unconscious patterns, of course. What we call "conscious" and what we call "unconscious" are merely different conditions, like being awake and being asleep. Both are basically beneficial if we allow them to be, despite the modern notion that consciousness is preferable in all ways and at all times. This popular ideal is at odds with reality because unconsciousness is as critical to our well-being as consciousness is. Indeed, unconsciousness may be one of the cleverer inventions of consciousness itself.

Much of what we call unconscious is information about ourselves and our functioning that we have learned so thoroughly, we have been able to take our attention away from it—to forget about it—and yet continue to know it. If you learned to ride a bicycle as a child, you can hop right on one twenty years later and pedal away without ever thinking about how to maintain your balance. You will always be able to ride a bicycle, and you need never think about how to do it again. Similarly, if you learned to walk in a relaxed and graceful manner, your body looks and feels balanced and you move with ease and fluidity: You need never think about walking again. If you learned to walk with tension and anxiety, however, your body looks and feels stiff, you move rigidly, and pain or discomfort will sooner or later force you to think about walking whenever you do it.

SEX AND THE UNCONSCIOUS BODY

One of the areas in which unconscious rigidities affect people most strongly is in their sexual functioning. At the slightest hint of arousal our glands begin to secrete their fluids, altering our physical and psychological makeup; several of our internal structures reposition themselves; and blood is redirected to our sex organs and other erogenous zones. As arousal increases the entire body prepares for this single act: Muscle tone increases, awareness of hunger and pain fade, and we become supremely sensitive to the unique sensations that overwhelm our bodies, literally from the hair follicles in our scalps to the muscles of our toes.

Unfortunately, most of us fail to feel nearly all these rich sensations and never know how much ecstasy is available to us. All we know is the gross buildup, the rush, and the genital orgasm. The reason is that we are too rigid to be aware of our own pleasure.

But as we become intimate with our bodies, our growing awareness keys us in to increasingly subtle levels of ecstasy, and we become vividly aware of the pleasure that has been awaiting us all along and that we have been missing.

Body awareness not only lets us enjoy more of the pleasure that is already present, it actually increases the amount of physical pleasure we can have in sex because it is accompanied by a relaxation of rigidity and tension throughout our bodies. As all movement becomes easier, stress and tension decrease, and ease and pleasure grow. Then sex, which is one of the most aerobic of all natural functions, becomes restorative instead of draining. This is another reason many people who have been through bodywork report vastly improved sexual lives.

Next time you are with your lover, see how far you can allow yourself to become conscious of the dance of sex. Forget the idea of controlling the action and seek instead the easy, flowing motions that are natural to your body. One cause of tension in sex is having the goal of orgasm; but orgasm will come when the time is right. With no goals in mind you can let your body relax. Your decreased effort will pay off in increased sexual pleasure.

FREE YOUR BODY, FREE YOURSELF

Early in his career, Sigmund Freud developed what was known as the "talking therapy" as a way to help people whose physical problems—such as rigidities and frigidity—seemed to him to derive from thoughts, feelings, and other experiences that had been repressed. He sought to treat his clients' bodies by using information from the unconscious parts of their minds. Ever since, therapies such as psychoanalysis and analytic psychology have used dreams, fantasies, and word-association responses to increase a person's awareness of those unconscious habits, processes, and connections that dominate his life. The therapist works with her client to elicit and analyze unconscious symbols and images, and as he becomes conscious of the material once again, the client becomes free to choose a course of living more satisfying than the one that brought him to therapy in the first place.

Just as our unconscious habits and beliefs affect our

21

bodies, so our bodily habits affect our minds. In structural bodywork the practitioner also enters his client's unconscious—though this is not the particular aim of the work —this time through the body. As he frees and realigns tight, misshapen muscles and allows them to assume their natural forms, the constricted patterns of mind that accompany physical rigidities also tend to relax. Once again, the client becomes increasingly able to choose a more satisfying way of being than the one that brought her to bodywork in the first place. As with any kind of learning, from walking to riding a bicycle to understanding the organization of one's own mind, the new, more flexible patterns gradually fade from consciousness to become part of the automaticity that allows us to live our lives freely.

ENERGY AND THE BODY

Let us say, as many people have before, that life is like a game of chess. If you are a piece on the chessboard and looking at the game in progress from that perspective, then your whole universe, everything that exists in your perception and in your imagination, is on that board. And if, from that vantage, you try to make sense of the game, you will find yourself highly frustrated. Your friends disappear off the board right and left without your having anything to say about it. What looks like a terrible defeat abruptly turns into a fantastic victory, and what looks like a fantastic victory is suddenly disclosed to be a horrible defeat, and as the game goes on all around you, you have no idea how long you're going to last on the board, or why. If you're a piece on the board the game looks all but nonsensical, and the reason is that there is one important element in the game that is *not* on the board, and whose absence you can not even perceive: the player. It is the player who makes sense of the game.

Since our chess game is a metaphor, let us extrapolate to what has been called the larger game of life. Trying to figure out life from the perspective of an individual alive on this planet doesn't make a lot of sense. Events occur without anyone having consulted you, great victories become defeats before your very eyes and vice versa, you have no idea how long you're going to last, and so forth. Once again, the confusion results from the absence of the decision maker, the sense maker, the player.

Over the course of history, we chess pieces have given the player various names, such as God, being, presence, essence, spirit, Self, energy. Energy is one way of naming something that exists beyond, but clearly manifests within, physical reality. It is what moves us, as the chess player moves the pieces on the board. Energy is the prime mover. Energy gives matter meaning. Energy by any other name is what we have called the unnameable, the unmentionable, that which was when all the worlds were without form, and void.

Einstein discovered that energy is ultimately identical with matter. While those of us who are neither mathematicians nor physicists may not understand the technical implications of his famous theories, it is clear nonetheless that our physical bodies and our essential energy are one and the same. Our bodies are our energy: It is through our bodies that we move.

THE GRAVITY OF THE SITUATION

We move in fields of forces, among the most pronounced of which is gravity. Gravity is an energetic force we cannot fail to feel. Yet, even though it affects us constantly, most of us never recognize its impact. Gravity is a force we discover in our first few years as we learn to move, to stand, to walk; then we forget about it, and pay it no further attention unless we're learning some new balancing act such as sailing or skiing or riding a bike. Unconsciously, though, we always know that gravity is with us. We dream of falling, of being earth-bound, of having solid ground beneath our feet; and we dream of being free of gravity, too: of flying, of winging it, of taking off.

To go unconscious is to lose track of your relationship with gravity. When you fall asleep, for instance, or when you are knocked out, you collapse physically as well as mentally. Since knowing anything about direction is a way of orienting yourself in the world, one aspect of consciousness is that it keeps you oriented in gravity: Consciousness, in a manner of speaking, is knowing which way is up.

The human body is well designed to function smoothly in the Earth's gravity. By nature we stand upright with virtually no effort; but when we are out of balance we strain against gravity, trying to hold ourselves in unnatural positions against its pull. That strain gradually constricts both our physical and our mental flexibilities.

In a mythic sense, perhaps this is why we hope crooks will go straight and turn themselves into upright citizens—because our social order is a macrosystem for us, as much as each of us is a macrosystem for the various principles organized within us. When people, places, and events get twisted beyond recognition around us, they not only serve to remind us of our own vulnerability but also point out for us the ways in which our larger systems may be out of whack.

THE BODY AS AN ENERGY PROCESSOR

Einstein proved that all matter is a form of energy; it follows then, that energy is a reflection of changes in the forms of matter. The prime function of the body's life support system is to process material incorporated from outside the body—food, water, air—and to extract energy from it for sustenance and growth. Our bodies also process other forms of energy as well, such as light, sound, and heat.

As an energy processor, the body reflects the holographic balance of a person's life: When the body and being are in balance we experience ease and grace; when they are dis-integrated we experience stress and pain.

Dis-integration of the body is often a sign that someone is simply unaware of herself as a physical presence —not that she is unaware of her physical *existence,* but that she is at odds with her body. A body that is out of alignment may be seen as a hologram that is out of focus: Its relationship with its energy source is blocked. But an imbalanced body is no disaster: From the point of view of structural integration, misalignment is a necessary step in a person's gaining the knowledge and insight that may permit her to *become* balanced. Recognition can be the start of a journey toward the natural state of ease, balance, and integration.

THE BODY BY DESIGN

The body's design function can be respected or abused either structurally or functionally. Structurally, for instance, if you are standing in a balanced posture you can breathe fully, filling your lungs as they are designed to be filled. On the other hand, if you slouch or stand at rigid attention, you compress your lungs so that they cannot operate as they are intended to. Functionally, no matter how adept your bellows movement may be, if you breathe air that is not composed of the balance of elements your body needs to survive, you can poison yourself or suffocate.

Like a hologram, your body is designed to process

particular energies in particular ways: You eat and breathe and walk upon the Earth within a specific range of balances. When the processing is in balance, so also is your life; when the processing is out of balance, so also is your life. Living a life of ease, balance, and integrity is not just a metaphor: It takes place literally, and is expressed in your bodily way of being in the world. It is a function of energy, and your body's design integrity is reflected in its success. When your body is in balance your whole life works better.

THE MIND AS AN INFORMATION PROCESSOR

The mind is analogous to the body in that, as the body processes energy, so the mind processes information. But the mind receives its raw information through the body, so distortions in the body lead inevitably to distortions in perception. Any imbalance results from operating the system in some way other than that for which it is designed.

Your body is also influenced by your beliefs and the ways in which you receive information from the world around you. For instance, if you think hot is cold or red is green you will attempt to function in a way your body's design cannot support. If you put your hand on a hot stove and interpret the resulting sensation as cool, you will burn yourself; if you think the traffic light has turned green when it has in fact turned red you are soon likely to have an accident.

Whether accurate or inaccurate, a belief is a function of the mind, and we express our minds in the world through our bodies all the time. When we interpret rigidity as strength, as many people do these days, we imply that it is weak to be flexible. If we then strive to be what we think of as strong, we make ourselves instead incapable of change; and that, in a world that is constantly

26

changing, is a progressive deterioration into the greatest weakness of all.

The mind and body are so intimately connected that ultimately we cannot tell the difference between them. Ultimately, indeed, they tell the same stories about us. But the body is the more visible aspect of the being and so may speak for the mind more eloquently than the mind can speak for itself. When we align the body we also align the mind. The body is the hologram of the being; and, as Alexander Lowen has said, "The body does not lie."

THE PLASTICITY OF THE HUMAN BODY

3

BIOFUNCTIONAL ANATOMY

To be plastic is to be flexible, pliable, renewable, and capable of changing without breaking. This is the way the human structure is designed to function. When we watch infants and children playing and exploring the boundaries of their worlds, it is obvious that plasticity is an inherent part of being human. But when we watch old people at their occupations, the suppleness of youth often seems to be gone, replaced by rigidity and stiffness. It is our common cultural assumption that such a progression is an inevitable concomitant of aging; but what if our assumption is wrong? What if, instead, the signs we ascribe to growing old result from misusing the bodies we started with until we are so overwhelmed by structural stress that we cease to be able to function comfortably? Until we wear them out and, part by part, turn their innate resilience into something brittle, fragile, and frail? What if, moreover, we could learn to use our bodies properly, in such a way that we might cease to do this damage to ourselves? And what if we could even *undo* some of the damage we've already done?

In this chapter we will examine some of the most important ways in which simple ignorance of the body's natural structure and functions can lead to dis-ease and disability. We will also see how understanding the body can allow us to be and to move with freedom and grace. We will not be concerned so much with understanding our bodies' technical anatomy and physiology, but rather with understanding anatomy in a biofunctional way: grasping the operational nature of how our bodies are integrated and how that integration makes the body as physically free as it is designed to be. We will also come to understand what we do—and can stop doing—that obstructs our freedom.

THE BODY AS A FLUID SYSTEM

One of the great misconceptions to which each of us has been educated is that the body is fundamentally a solid object. This teaching is not so much explicit as it is implied by the ways in which we describe and talk about the body in Western culture, and the way we finally come to think of it as an interlocking system of gears, levers, pulleys, and plates—as a machine, in brief. Perhaps the error of our ways is due to the great success of the Industrial Revolution, which surrounded us with machinery we came to identify as extensions of ourselves, and in which we came to see ourselves reflected. Or perhaps people in the late 18th and the 19th centuries already thought of the body mechanically, and the existing understanding enabled the great inventors of that era to conceive of their machines as superbly sturdy flesh that required neither vacations nor fringe benefits. However it came about, even some modern anatomy and kinesiology textbooks still describe the human body and its movements in terms of solid structures and solid mechanics. While this sort of metaphor makes for rich literature, it is simply not accurate. The human body is not a solid system at all. In fact, it contains hardly any parts that can be remotely understood as solid.

Depending on the individual and the moment in his or her life, the human body is composed of between 50 and 65 percent water. It is no surprise, then, that the majority of its elements are fluid filled. Even the bones, the body's most solid components, are filled with liquid marrow; and virtually everything else, from the muscles to the organs to the nerves, is composed of fluid-filled sacs, pumps, and semipermeable membranes constantly crossed by flowing fluids.

When you imagine the body in mechanical terms, you may easily think of a muscle as a kind of rubber band attached to a bone, which lengthens when you pull it and gets shorter when you let it go. But a truer description of a muscle is of a fluid-filled bag that contracts and expands in two ways: First, by changing shape under externally imposed pressure, as a balloon does when you squeeze it; and second, by releasing and acquiring fluids across membrane walls, to and from the tissues around it, in the processes of tightening and relaxing.

Fluidity is a willingness or ability to change, while rigidity is resistance to change. Resistance to change is a highly desirable quality in a material such as steel, because we rely on its ability to maintain its shape when we put it to use. But it is not so desirable in water, whose strength lies in its ability to follow the path of least resistance, conforming readily to the shape of whatever container may hold it at any moment.

A system based on fluid mechanics moves in a different way than does a system based on solid mechanics. It moves like a river, or a cat, or tall grass in a breeze, instead of like pistons and cogged wheels. Implicit in this difference is that a fluid system has a wider latitude of movement available to it—more possibilities for more different kinds of movement in more directions under more varied circumstances—than a mechanical system has. It is this latitude that is expressed in its greater flexibility.

As with any other system, the more we human beings are rigid the less we are liable to change, and the more we are fluid the more we are adaptable. Since life is a process of continual change, fluidity is usually the more successful state. In psychological terms, for example, fluidity suggests the ability to move from anger to sorrow to affection to joy as appropriate to the moment and situation, without becoming stuck in any one condition. The emotionally healthy person has a whole spectrum of psychic movement available. Something similar is true for the physically healthy person: Open and able to change, he has a wide field of bodily movement available. In all dimensions, the more rigidity prevails, the less movement is possible.

Being available to change does not imply flaccidity, however. The body is normally organized to provide a stable structure by including elements that span a continuum from the rigidity of bones to the fluidity of water. The health of the structure is seen in its balance between the poles of flexibility and stability, in which the organism can be sufficiently adaptable to change when change is appropriate, without relinquishing its basic structure. Bodily changes take place, then, within a framework designed to accommodate them.

The human body is not unique in its fluidity, of course. Fluidity is a quality of all living organisms, and it may very well be considered the *sine qua non* of life itself. From the cellular level on up, water is the molecular element common to living things on Earth. Life as we know it was born from water, it migrated out onto land

Water—the ace of elements. Water dives from the clouds without parachute, wings or safety net. Water runs over the steepest precipice and blinks not a lash. Water is buried and rises again; water walks on fire and fire gets the blisters. Stylishly composed in any situation—solid, gas or liquid—speaking in penetrating dialects understood by all things—animal, vegetable or mineral—water travels intrepidly through four dimensions, *sustaining* (Kick a lettuce in the field and it will yell "Water!"), *destroying* (The Dutch boy's finger remembered the view from Ararat) and *creating* (It has even been said that human beings were invented by water as a device for transporting itself from one place to another, but that's another story).

Always in motion, ever-flowing (whether at steam rate or glacier speed), rhythmic, dynamic, ubiquitous, changing and working its changes, a mathematics turned wrong side out, a philosophy in reverse, the ongoing odyssey of water is virtually irresistible.
—Tom Robbins, *Even Cowgirls Get the Blues*

in the forms of fish and vegetation, and to this day every living substance on Earth is a package of water, needing water to maintain its survival. Perhaps it is no wonder, then, that all living things are characterized by their fluid flow; that within the range of their peculiar structures they express their health by the greatest possible fluidity.

The process of life may be seen as one in which we start out 99 percent water and end up virtually solid. It may be seen as a process of drying up, or drying out, or being hung up to dry. The Bible says dust to dust, but physiologically our process is water to dust. We each begin as a single cell, the fertilized egg, that is almost entirely fluid. By the time we're adults our bodies have become more than one-third solid; and when we die, all our bodily fluids evaporate and our bodies dessicate.

In the course of aging, most of us find ourselves increasingly sedentary and confined, moving less and less. We may claim our static state results from pain, fatigue, or laziness, but which, in fact, comes first? To function properly, the body relies heavily on the movement of fluids, and as rigidity sets in the fluid flow is impaired. It is no wonder that many diseases of aging are related to circulatory problems: Arteriosclerosis, embolisms, impaired bowel function, and blocked lymphatic drainage, for example, are all conditions that in one way or another reflect the degeneration of fluid flow. The resulting characteristic is that of becoming wizened and sere—of drying up.

We tend to put sick people to bed. The rationale for this form of treatment is that bed rest conserves energy, leaving the body's resources available to combat its disease. For certain ailments, such as large-scale infections, this makes eminently good sense; but for illnesses that are more mechanical than systemic, bed rest only frees up energy that has no outlet, while the body's tissues begin to stagnate from lack of movement. People with arthritis, for example, report that they feel worst in the mornings, when they first wake up. As they start to move about, their rigidity and pain tend to dissipate.

The Yiddish word *zaftig,* which literally means "juicy," is applied to full-bodied people, usually in the prime of their lives. This vivid image reflects something of a subconscious understanding that we are healthiest when we are most like mature fruit—ripe and full. Then, as we pass our prime, we move from plum to prune; and we perceive older people that way, as wrinkled and dried up. There is no shame in aging, but it is not necessary to *suffer* aging as much as most of us do, and it is possible to extend the duration of the juicy, fruitful years by encouraging the fluidity of our physical structures. Although we can help ourselves by being attentive to all the aspects of our lives, a fine first way is to encourage movement.

MOVEMENT

We admire a skilled dancer, skier, or skater not only for her strength and grace but especially for the fluidity of her movement. Perhaps this is because we have forgotten, and she reminds us, that we are fluid too.

With the exception of the circulatory system, whose fluid movement is maintained by the heart, none of the body's specifically fluid systems has an independent pump. Instead, it is the ordinary movement of common, everyday activities that keeps the body's juices flowing, as it is their flowing that enables us to move. Even when you are at rest you move by breathing, and that movement is disseminated throughout your structure by the very fluids the movement moves. All the shifting around that is one of life's constants takes place at every level of the organism, from the microscopic cell to the macroscopic body.

Our concern in this section is the movement of the whole human structure, rather than, say, the movement of a single cell or the circulation of fluids between the tissues. Movement, as we will consider it here, means movement of the body—moving in normal human activities.

THE BODY IN MOTION

Movement is a principal body function, integrally involved in the expression of everything we do and everything we are. If some people seem to move too little, so that their very *ability* to move atrophies, other people seem to move too much, as if they cannot contain themselves. There is no hard-and-fast rule that stipulates what constitutes too much or too little movement. A person who is merely taking a slow stroll around the block is moving too much if, at the same time, she is asleep. By the same token, a person is moving too little if he is ambling along at the same sort of leisurely pace while crossing a busy freeway.

The degree of movement that is appropriate and healthy varies not only with the situation one is in, but also with the part of the body in question. For instance, the knee has appropriate movement of about 150 degrees in the single plane from front to back, which allows it to act as the stable hinge between the levers of the shin and thigh. Lateral movement, or movement 360 degrees front to back, would be excessive for the knee because either would destabilize the structure, just as a maximum range of 10 degrees front to back would be inadequate to allow it to fulfill its function.

The limits and freedom of movement that exist for the knee have their counterparts with respect to every system of the body. When the limits become too rigid for some body part, its freedom is diminished, as you can feel for yourself by trying the following exercise.

Without changing the position you are now in, whether sitting, standing, or lying down, tighten your leg muscles. Keeping them tight, tighten your abdomen. Maintaining this grip on your lower body, tighten your chest, arms, shoulders, and neck. Now, breathe: In, out. In, out. In, out. How does it feel? In, out. In, out. Although the condition is exaggerated, the experience of breathing you are now having is fundamentally the one most people have most of the time. In, out. In, out. Is it any wonder that we often feel stressed and anxious, and that our work and our relationships have a strained quality to them? In, out. In, out. Where is our freedom of movement when we are locked into a pattern of rigidity we may not even know exists? Now, relax all those muscles, from your feet up, and then breathe again. In, out. In, out. This is the sort of change in the body's holding patterns that leads to living a life of ease.

As with the knee, the proper movement of any structure is best determined by looking at its design function. The design function of a wind sock at the airport is to indicate the wind's direction and approximate force at any given moment, and its proper movement constantly reflects the slightest change in wind direction and velocity. The design functions of the mouth are to ingest and chew food, and to give form to our vocal sounds. But design function can be altered by inappropriate use. Consider the wind sock with a large rock stitched into its gullet, or your mouth if it is perpetually clamped shut in tension or anger. Their structures have been so changed that they can no longer perform their original functions properly. Either their structures must be changed once more, or their functions must be redefined in order to make them useful again.

THE LEARNING BODY

Our bodies are naturally designed to enable us to move gracefully and efficiently, yet many of us learn movement patterns early in life that impede our physical functioning. If you have the opportunity to stand behind three generations of a family while they walk, especially if all three people are of the same gender, you are likely to see the phenomenon of family movement traits in action. John Smith, Jr., moves in a manner identifiably like his father's, and his son moves much as he does. Therefore, we may say, "That's John Smith's boy: You can tell by the way he walks." But even if his physical structure is radically different from that of his relatives, young John's movements may be as much his father's as they are his own. That is, his movement (function) may be as appropriate for the design of his father's body (structure) as it is for his own. Why?

John Smith, Jr., demonstrates that we human beings *learn* to move. When we are children beginning to walk we learn through a great deal of trial and error. At first, of course, our trials are mostly error; but as our walking is increasingly successful, our error rate diminishes until it is small enough that we achieve the results we seek: We can get where we want to go on our own two feet without falling or even stumbling very often. Thereafter, we repeat our achievement over and over again until it becomes habit.

The habits of movement we develop when we are children include our errors. These may not be obvious errors such as falling and stumbling, which we overcome in time, but other errors less apparent in the light of our successes, such as imperfect balance. We correct these kinds of errors with counterbalancing muscle tension and effort, incorporating both the error *and the error inherent in its correction* in the way we move for the rest of our lives.

Watch yourself in a mirror as you walk, and you can begin to see the child you were, protected by the adult you have become. If you were afraid of falling forward as a little kid, you may have developed the habit of holding your shoulders back as a form of compensation. Consequently, as an adult your habitual posture may lead you to walk with your weight on your heels, creating unnecessary strain on your spine, and you may compensate in turn for the added strain by thrusting your head forward. With this posture you actually *increase* your chances of falling forward, but by now your habit is ingrained. Similarly, you may have been afraid of being attacked, and learned to walk with your shoulders hunched forward and up for protection. Now, twenty or thirty or forty years later, you may find your shoulders still held high, crunching your neck so that you get headaches, and pulling on your rib cage so that you cannot draw a full breath.

These sorts of disabilities, which most of us do not even recognize, are not irreversible: They only feel that way when we first become aware of the pain, stress, and fatigue they have caused us every minute of our adult lives.

We also learn by imitation. Little John, from our example above, looks around to find out how the other members of his tribe get from place to place, and he tries to do what they do. Especially he tries to emulate the people he loves, admires, and identifies with, such as his father. And again, as he grows up, he gets the hang of things: Not only can he walk without falling, he can also walk like John, Sr.

If John Smith, Sr., walks with *his* shoulders high, John, Jr., is likely to do the same, even if the circumstances of his life suggest no reason for such a posture. Ida Rolf used to show a short film clip of a father and son walking away from the camera in which the father, who had suffered a war injury, walked with a slight limp. The son, who was seven or eight years old, walked with exactly the same limp, even though there was no reason in his structure for the limp to be present. The child was building into his body all the problems inherent in a limp by imitating the limp in the first place. Of course, he didn't think of it as imitating, or as perpetuating inefficiency, or as building up a condition of imbalance. But he will pay the price of his misalignment in stressed muscles and disproportionately weighted bones and all their attendant ills for the rest of his life. Whose movement habits have you embodied? And where did those people pick them up in the first place?

Learning goes on past childhood, so we continue to have the opportunity to pick up all kinds of habits that may cause us pain and stress. We pick up attitudes about movement and posture not only from our families but also from television and advertising images of some mythic ideal physique, from our own individual psychologies, and in response to physical trauma, such as when we favor a leg broken in a football game until the opposing hip is chronically raised and shifts the bulk of our weight to a single foot that grows calloused and crooked from the imbalance. We have *all* adopted some movements that do not function well for us, and that exact a price from us in terms of dis-ease, imbalance, pain, discomfort, and a distorted physical integrity.

One apparent solution to our physical ailments is to train our bodies to function according to the structures we have developed. This is actually what most of us have done without realizing it. Our pelvises stick out, making us look thick in the waist and loose in the seat, so we buy books and attend classes that are supposed to make our stomachs flatter, our buttocks tighter, our chests larger, or our waists smaller—that is, to make us even more like some other image of who we are supposed to be, and even less like ourselves than we already are.

But not every body is created to look like whatever popular symbols of masculinity or femininity are currently in vogue. If, instead of trying to be someone else, we each simply accepted our own inherent physical designs, we could eliminate most of the struggle and effort that seem to go along with trying to stay fit.

MOVING IN BALANCE

Perhaps you can recall how, when you were a child, you practiced balancing a stick on the tip of your finger. Imagine that you are doing so again now. When that stick is at the balance point, it can fall in any direction; but if the stick is out of balance, it can fall only one way. Similarly, when you are standing on your feet, in balance, not leaning in any direction and at rest, you are capable of your maximum movement potential: Within the constraints of your body's structure, you can move equally well in any direction. But when you are out of balance, all possibilities are gone except the one specific direction in which you are already inclined.

Just as the stick that is leaning can fall in only one direction, so also your body, if it is predisposed to some particular direction, can only fall that way—or, more precisely, in order to move in some other direction it requires that you exert additional effort of will and of body. If you do not want to fall, you must exercise that effort just to stand up. You thereby create an imbalance on top of the preexisting imbalance, and you have to expend yet more energy to accomplish what may appear to you to be nothing more than standing in one place. The following exercise will give you a sense of what this means.

Holding this book in your hands, stand up and bend over to one side, from the waist. If you can bend your body to a 90-degree angle without discomfort, do so; otherwise, bend over to the side as far as comfort will allow. Now, stay in that position while you read this exercise. Or stay, at least, until your discomfort level prompts you to stand up while the standing is good. You may be surprised at the length of time you can maintain this unusual posture—not because you will be able to do it for long, but precisely because you will not.

If you are still bent over by the time you reach this sentence, try walking around the room in your new position until you have a clear sense of just how it is that unbalanced structure can affect your functioning. In particular, watch for the ways you start to compensate for your imbalance that you might have thought had nothing to do with reading, bending, or walking—the way you tense your neck and shoulders, for instance, or the way your breathing grows ragged, or the way you have begun to tighten your thighs, and plant your feet and grip the ground with your toes.

Your muscles are showing you exactly how you have used stress to hide *all* your bodily imbalances from yourself. If you were forced by a cast or a brace to walk like this for a few hours, you would find it difficult to stand upright again when the restraint was removed. If you were forced to walk like this for a few weeks you might spend days straightening yourself out. And if you were forced to walk like this for ten or twenty or thirty years, you might never get straight again. In fact, you might come to feel that this position was your natural one, and that an upright posture was painfully unnatural.

Whatever ways you have been maintaining imbalances in your life—particularly if they took root before you were aware that there was any alternative—now feel proper to you. But they are imposing stress on your body just as standing bent over to the side has stressed it. This is why true freedom of movement leads to a life of ease and balance. If you are still bent over, stand up now—if you can.

Balance is a state of equilibrium. When the stick is leaning in any direction, it has no choice but to fall because there is nothing to hold it up. People are not sticks, of course. We can lean without falling, but only through constant exertion. Our effort results in something that resembles balance insofar as we are not falling over, but it is really a resistance to falling over, which, as we have seen, demands effort and is restricting. This is something quite different from balance.

What most of us think of as balance is this sort of state of contraction, of holding things together so they will not fall apart. Over time, this sort of posture becomes habitual, and it results in chronic rigidity. Thus, our traditional picture of balance is the scales, poised and standing still between two extremes. But this is an inaccurate picture of balance and of the scales: The picture is of a moment fixed in a time long past. In reality, equally weighted and balanced scales sway constantly, gently, and gracefully about their middle point. If you remove the weight from one side of the scales, they *do* achieve a static state: They fall *klunk* over to one side and stop—which is exactly the picture of *im*balance. The tightrope walker falls if he tries to stand still; he must be in motion all the time. When you learn to ride a bicycle you do not learn to maintain a static line, but to fall and correct your fall, from side to side, constantly and rapidly, achieving thereby a condition of balance. Balance is not a static condition, but a process of constant flux, a fluid expression of wholeness and ease.

Because imbalanced movement is generally mechanical rather than fluid, it is often destructive rather than helpful in a living body. A mechanical analogy is that when your car's wheels are misaligned, driving and turning them more will not improve matters; in fact, until you realign them, further movement will only increase the damage being done to your vehicle. Invariably, appropriate function can be discerned in an entity's design structure, and in the awareness that function follows form as surely as form follows function.

MOVEMENT AND AGING

Most people think the process of aging is a function of the passage of time. If by "aging" we mean "adding years," this is accurate. But if we mean developing the physical attributes of wrinkles, a stoop, and general decrepitude, it is not.

The process that is commonly seen as aging is partly a function of losing fluidity, as we have observed. But it is also a function of the accumulation of tension and rigidity in the tissues of the body. In our world, tension and stress are realities; they impinge upon our bodies all the time. When we ignore these pressures or pretend they do not affect us, we are prone to absorb them into our physical forms, which is why your personal levels of tension and stress rise when you are out of touch with— unaware of—your body.

In order to minimize the effects of aging, it is useful to cease paying attention to the passage of time and to start paying attention to your bodily holding patterns, to the ways in which stress, tension, and pain appear in your person. For example, most people think that wrinkles come with increasing age. So notice, as you read this paragraph, whether you are wrinkling your forehead or squeezing your eyebrows together in an effort to see and understand what is in front of you. Go to your mirror and reproduce the expression you've been using to concentrate and see how old you think you look. Now, close your eyes and place the palms of your hands over your face so that your fingertips meet your hairline. Slowly smooth out your face by bringing your hands down your cheeks and jowls, wiping out any expression you may be wearing. Open your eyes again and see how many years you've lost in your face.

To lose some years in your body, too, stand in front of the mirror and slouch or stoop. Do it some more. Get into it, and slouch the way you think old people are supposed to slouch. This exercise is not difficult, because your slouching posture will only be an exaggeration of what you brought to the mirror in the first place. Imagine that there is a hook in your ceiling. Picture it descending until it hovers right above the base of your neck. Now, let that hook lift you so that the rest of your body just hangs from the hook like a suit of clothes. How many years have you lost in your body? There is no reason an old person cannot stand as straight as you are now, or straighter. As you grow old, you do not have to be dragged to the ground.

MOVEMENT AS EXERCISE AND FITNESS

Movement is good for the body as a general rule, and many people undertake some form of movement as exercise and as a way to keep fit. But movement performed with effort instead of ease—especially rigorous movement—builds rigidities that undermine its benefits by damaging the body structure.

The dangers of frequent, long-duration running, including shin splints, fallen arches, hip displacements, and torn cartilages and ligaments, have been well documented. They appear as signs of physical damage, or of stress verging on distress, not because running is bad for the body but because in movement tension acts like friction. When combined with structural imbalances, it demands efforts from the body that the body is not designed to accomplish. In other words, if your body is already structurally imbalanced, exercise will make it *worse,* not better.

To gain maximum benefits from exercise it is necessary not only to move, but to move gracefully. This is accomplished by learning to relax through the movement itself, as the martial arts teach but calisthenic exercises usually do not. Finally, though, the issue is not which activity you prefer, but how you go about doing it.

The indispensible step in turning exercise movements into fitness movements is to pay attention to those signals the body communicates as pain. It is not necessary to stop most exercises that hurt, but to prevent damage it may be essential to modify them so that they cease to be painful: To stop trying so hard, and find an easy, balanced way to accomplish your goal.

Balance means different things in different forms of exercise. In tennis, for example, where a player turns a great deal around the body's axis at the shoulders and ankles, one kind of imbalance, displayed as improper positioning of the arm and racquet, results in tennis elbow. The simplest solution to tennis elbow is to consult a professional tennis coach who can teach you to hold the racquet properly. Meanwhile, a physical therapist can relieve immediate pain in your arm. If you ignore the pain you will not only suffer needlessly in the present, but you will instigate a cycle of increasing rigidity in your arm and shoulder that will soon involve your whole body. Not only will tennis cease to be fun, but any strenuous exercise at all may become uncomfortable.

In aerobics, the difference between lumbering like an ox and prancing like a deer is a matter of being light on your feet; being light on your feet is a matter of being in balance. When you do an aerobics workout out of balance, you impose your body weight repeatedly on muscles, tendons, ligaments, and bones, compressing your spine and joints, provoking lower-back pains and ailments similar to those that runners suffer. Performed in balance and easily, aerobics can stretch your body and make you limber, while providing the cardiovascular workout you want.

If you swim with your head up, your shoulders and neck will tire quickly. The solution is simply to relax and get your face wet. Again, unless you are swimming competitively or for speed, there is no reason to swim hard. The fluid element of water rewards ease with more ease, as well as with increased efficiency.

Fitness is not simply a matter of getting exercise. It is the sum of many factors, including diet, rest, and a life whose elements are in harmony with each other. From the bodyworker's point of view, it is vastly harder to be fit if your structure is *not* well-aligned than if it is. Before taking any rigorous exercise be sure to stretch and warm up properly. Approaching your workout loose and limber is one critical step to exercise fitness. It is also the beginning of awareness: the start of a process through which you can become increasingly sensitive to lesser degrees of pain and discomfort in your body, so that you can take effective action for it.

THE BODY AS STRUCTURE AND FUNCTION

In the human body, as everywhere else, structure determines function, and function affects structure. To some degree, the plasticity of the body allows structures that have highly specific purposes to develop in response to the demands placed upon them. This ability is present in most of the body's parts, but nowhere is it so apparent as in the tissue known as the *mesoderm*. Mesoderm, which we will discuss at greater length in this chapter's next section, includes all the tissue we commonly refer to as muscle, and it is especially responsive to demand. When we increase our use of most muscles, they grow larger; when we decrease their use, they grow smaller. To some extent, then, our bodies reshape themselves according to the way we use them. This ability is a great tribute to the adaptability of the organism; it also suggests why fluid habits of movement induce a flexible body and why stiff habits of movement can result in a rigid, unresponsive body.

Further, the body's regenerative ability tends to obscure some of the damage it sustains until it has accumulated enough to burst into our consciousness as disease, pain, and stress. This is the reason many people go along in their lives feeling that everything is okay until suddenly, at the age of twenty or thirty or forty or more, they start waking up with back pain, arthritis, or some other expression of muscular or skeletal strain. To most of us, the appearance of such distress seems abrupt, an eruption with no prior history or symptom. But the obvious damage is only the visible part of a process that has been going on for years.

Consider the common garden hose. If you connect it to a spigot, close off its nozzle, and turn on the water, the hose will eventually burst in one spot or another. Looking at the situation rationally, you may conclude that the problem was a weak spot in the rubber tubing. But what you have identified is the symptom, not the problem. The problem is that too much pressure built up in the hose, and the hose gave out.

Continuing to place stress on the structures of our bodies is just like continuing to force water into the closed-off hose. The pressure overload may pass unnoticed until the problem explodes through one of the structure's weakened points. By balancing our body's structure with its functioning we can minimize the chances that it will be subjected to some sort of breakdown. Appropriate movement is the key to such balance, but for nearly everyone, learning to move in a balanced manner cannot occur until the physical structure has first been returned to a condition of balance.

THE BODY AS A TENSEGRITY STRUCTURE

Many people conceive of the skeleton as a rigid framework holding up the body from the center, with everything else sort of hanging from the bones. Perhaps we have come to think of the body this way as a result of watching tall office buildings go up all over the land. We see that those buildings start out as rigid steel frameworks bolted and welded together, and that floors, ceilings, walls, elevator shafts, air conditioning vents, facing, and everything else needed to complete the building are attached to its framework. We even refer to the steel structure as the building's skeleton; we talk about its facing as the building's skin, and we call its mechanical core its heart, or, sometimes, its guts. But our animalian, or even anthropomorphic, view of a building's structure is simply an example of misplaced analogy, attractive and easy to use, but entirely inaccurate.

When you look at the human skeleton some physicians and other body professionals keep in their offices, you see that its parts are all held together by wires and bolts. If they were not, that skeleton would be nothing but a pile of bones. In other words, within the body itself, where there are no wires and bolts, the bones do not just hang together like the welded beams of some great building. They are kept in place some other way. They are maintained in their proper positions by soft tissue, which means that, contrary to the popular view, it is the rest of the body that holds the bones in place.

The implication of this observation, first advanced by Ida Rolf in her book, *Rolfing: The Integration of Human Structure,* is that the bones are spacers, whose function in terms of the body's structure is to determine the proper distance between its various parts, and to make certain that that spacing is not compromised. For instance, the bone in your upper arm, called the humerus, maintains a constant distance between your elbow and your shoulder. Without the humerus your randomly placed elbow might rub against your shoulder for awhile, then move to the level of your bicep, drop down toward your lower arm, and return to any which place. Would this be an odd way for an arm to function?

No, not really, although it would be an odd way for *your* arm to function. An octopus tentacle behaves in just this way. It is a jointless limb, capable of bending in any place while remaining highly viable. Its structure is appropriate to its function in a totally fluid environment. But your joints are very specifically located, appropriate to your upright functions on land. Each of those joints is nothing more than space filled with liquid across which two bones are held in place by straps known as ligaments. The space allows the bones to move, the ligaments help to define the parameters of their movement, and the bones, by defining the placement and even the function of the flesh around them, define the nature of the movement itself.

The concept of the bones as spacers in the body, contained and held together by soft tissue, is clearly and accurately represented in a model advanced by Buckminster Fuller, which he calls a *tensegrity structure*. The word *tensegrity* is a contraction of "tensional integrity." In order to understand its application properly, we should have some comprehension of two simple terms used by engineers to explain certain structural conditions.

Tension results from things being pulled apart. During a tug-of-war, when two people are pulling the two ends of a rope in opposite directions, the rope is in tension. A force along its length is pulling the two ends of the rope away from its middle. The cables from which the Golden Gate Bridge is suspended are under tension, pulled apart by the weight of the hanging bridge.

Compression is tension's exact opposite, and results from things being pressed together. When you lean on a cane, the cane is compressed between the floor and the weight of your body. A force at each of its two ends presses the length of the cane together toward its middle. Another example: When you squeeze an accordion, you are compressing it.

The word *tension* is commonly used to mean what

an engineer means by "compression." When we say, for example, that some tissues in the body are tense, an engineer would understand them to be compressed. If you stand up now and bend over to your right, then your right side is compressed, while your left side is tensed. Similarly, when we speak about states of psychological stress, we often say we are tense, whether we actually feel we are bearing the effects of pressure (compression) or feel that we are being pulled in different directions (tension).

Until Buckminster Fuller came along, virtually every structure human beings had built was compressional in nature, meaning that its integrity—its wholeness, what held it together—was based in its compressional elements: The hard pieces were in contact with each other, with force pressing them together in a way that allowed the structure to be maintained. For instance, the wall of a house is compressed by the ceiling, with which it is in contact. The ceiling itself is compressed by its own weight and by the resistance of the wall, and passes this compression to the other walls with which it is also in contact. The whole of the house presses on its foundation, and the foundation presses the ground on which the house stands. The continuity of the entire structure exists through compressional elements touching one another.

In a tensegrity structure, on the other hand, the integrity and continuity of the unit is based in its tensional elements: Strings or wires or other sorts of lines connect with each other under the force of continual tension maintained by the hard pieces of the structure—its compressional elements—which do not touch each other at all; they exist simply as spacers, maintaining the proper degree of tension in the structure as a whole by keeping the compressional elements at the proper distances from each other.

It is difficult at first to visualize the way a tensegrity

structure works, because neither nature nor human inge-
nuity provided us with any easily recognized referents
until Fuller built his models. A balloon offers some sense
of tensegrity if you think of its skin as the structure's
tensional element and air as its compressional element,
but it is not quite a satisfactory example because the
entire compressional element gives way when the tensional element is violated at any point—in other words,
the balloon bursts when you prick it with a pin—which
is not the case with a true tensegrity structure. A geodesic
dome, continued beneath the ground on which it rests
until it becomes spherical, also gives some sense of a
tensegrity structure's form, except that it is made of hard
pieces that compress each other. When we seek an example, the important feature of a true tensegrity structure
is that its continuity exists through elements under tension, and its compressional elements, its hard pieces,
exist as spacers to maintain that tension.

If the human body were a true compressional structure, the skull would press on the upper vertebrae of the
spine, the shoulders and clavicles would press on the
sternum and compress the rib cage, the whole upper
body would press down on the pelvis and lower back,
and everything would weigh down through the legs to
press the feet heavily against the earth. Running, skipping,
and jumping for joy would not likely be in the realm of
human experience. If this description of the body as a
compressional structure reminds you somewhat of your
own experience, it is possible that the flexibility and freedom of movement you do have is what you have settled
for, and is far less than you are capable of.

As a tensegrity structure, however, the muscles, skin,
and particularly the connective tissues connect with each
other under the tension of being kept separate, while the
body's hard compressional elements, the bones, maintain the structure of the tensional elements by keeping

them in their places where they will never touch each other. (Or should not: A rubbing together of two bones will produce agonizing pain, and signals a structural problem of great severity.)

The human body is designed to be a true tensegrity structure. The connective tissues are the body's organ of structure; the muscles are the tensioners of these membranes, and the bones, kept separate from one another by the fluid-filled space of the joints, maintain sufficient tension on the compressional muscles and connective tissue envelopes to keep them properly spaced.

The tensegrity structure is enormously economical. It provides more strength with less material than other support structures do, and it distributes stress evenly throughout the structure rather than allowing it to become concentrated at one or a few points where its accumulation is most likely to damage the structure's integrity. It also provides both more stability *and* more flexibility, using less-rigid materials, than compressional structures can offer.

It is only when the body becomes misaligned that the tensegrity structure collapses into a compressional mode, leading to all the accumulated stresses we associate with the aging process. The alignment that is critical to maintenance of the human tensegrity structure is essentially vertical; and our vertical alignment is the result of an organizing line around which this tensegrity structure can form itself.

VERTICAL ALIGNMENT

The human body's nearly complete organization around a vertical line is unique in the animal kingdom,* and it carries with it decided advantages and disadvantages.

*Birds are not in their true element when they walk on two legs: Their structure is adapted for horizontal flight. The great apes, on the other hand, can stand on their hind limbs but are better adapted to crouching, using their forelimbs to provide both balance and support.

The chief disadvantage is instability. The average human body is about five feet, six inches high and weighs 150 pounds. This structure rests on two platforms that together cover an area less than one foot square, a large portion of which does not even come into direct contact with the ground. That is a remarkably small base of support for an organism of such a size.

Three advantages offset the human structure's instability. First, bipedal vertical alignment provides us with far more rotational mobility than any other animal enjoys. Second, it gives us a higher center of gravity than most four-legged animals have. And third, it frees our forelimbs —our arms—from the task of locomotion. It is a quite traditional supposition that this last advantage, a freedom that is directly related to our being vertically rather than horizontally aligned, has contributed to the development of civilization and technology in all its facets.

When we look at the human being's vertical alignment, we see its mass dominated by a trunk. At the bottom of the trunk there is a bony support structure called the pelvis, which is a sort of bowl supporting the trunk's internal contents. Attached to this pelvic bowl are the two legs that reach down, and a vertical rod known as the spine that reaches up. At the top of the trunk is a girdle or yoke from which the arms depend. The spinal rod travels through that yoke, and the head rests on top of it.

A few pages back, when we were discussing movement, we talked about balancing a stick on the tip of your finger when you were a child. You may recall now that when the stick was perfectly vertical you could keep it upright with no effort at all, but as soon as it tilted the slightest degree, you had to expend a great deal of energy running back and forth and waving your arm about in order to keep it from falling over altogether.

Learning to align our bodies with gravity is not unlike learning to align that stick, because gravity provides the line around which the human structure organizes itself. And the origin of any structure's stresses and supports lies in its relationship with gravity: Gravity is the teacher, the organizing principle.

Looking at the human body, which is as close to home as we can come, we find that when we behave in accordance with our own design, we actually *seek* to be vertical, and gravity supports our attempt: We do not fall over, and standing upright requires no special effort. When we behave otherwise, however, gravity becomes our stressor: We can maintain our verticality only through enormous strain.

For example, if you have a pain in the bottom of your right foot, you may favor that foot by putting more of your weight on your left foot. Your left foot then becomes the repository of entirely new tensions that have nothing to do with your original pain, but do throw your body further out of balance. By this time you are having to exert considerable effort to stand upright, because most of your weight is on your left foot and gravity is therefore tugging at your left side. In order to remain upright you are compressing your right side; in the process you are squeezing the spaces between your bones—your joints— creating entirely new pains and physical distortions. In time, if this symphony of competing stresses cannot be alleviated, your whole body literally changes shape to accommodate your tilt to the left. When we resist gravity we seek to be free of stress through effort rather than ease, and instead of a vertically balanced, integrated body, we end up with something radically imbalanced and out of joint.

It would be nice if we could simply return our bodies to their inherent states of balance as easily as we return them to sitting positions after we have been standing. Unfortunately, we are intertwined with our imbalances, stresses, and tensions. We cannot affect one part of the body without affecting all the others. For this reason, true vertical alignment is achieved most easily and with least effort once we have already found our balance. In realigning ourselves we generally need a little help from the outside. This, of course, is where structural bodywork comes in. In the next section of this chapter we'll take a look at the body's biofunctional structure and begin to see what that structure is and how bodywork affects it.

ECTODERM, ENDODERM, AND MESODERM

Understanding the developmental origins of our various body systems can help us understand their structures and functions in our lives. It can also help us understand why different sorts of bodywork have different effects on us.

We know that we each began life as a single fertilized cell, and that as this cell reproduced it diversified into many different kinds of cells, which eventually became our arms, legs, internal organs, and so forth. It is in the second week of fetal life that a circle of cells called the embryonic disc forms two distinct layers, known as the endoderm and the ectoderm; by the sixteenth day a third germ layer, the mesoderm, appears between them. Although all three of these germ layers emerge from the original single cell, their purposes are quite distinct, and they become increasingly differentiated as the embryo grows.

The *ectoderm,* for instance, which is the outer layer of undifferentiated cell, becomes the skin, hair, nails, tooth enamel, mammary glands, and nervous system; its primary functions pertain to the body's ability to communicate both internally and externally. The *endoderm* is the inner germ layer, principally concerned with converting various materials in the environment into the kinds of energy the body requires for its survival and well-being. The endoderm becomes the guts: the gastrointestinal tract, the liver, pancreas, bladder, lungs, and trachea. The

The Sheldon Somatotypes

Over the millennia, philosophers and scientists of every stamp have sought to understand human temperament through the body's form. Twenty-five hundred years ago Hippocrates, the Father of Medicine, posited that people could be classified according to the humor, or body fluid, that most influenced their characters. The Choleric person, dominated by yellow liver bile, would be bilious and quick to anger; the Melancholic person, dominated by black bile, would be sad and depressed; the Phlegmatic person, dominated by phlegm, would be cool and calm even to the point of being sluggish and apathetic; while the Sanguine person, dominated by the blood, would be cheerful, confident, and optimistic. We still use these adjectives today to describe those sorts of character traits.

In the 15th century, the Swiss physician Paracelsus suggested there might be more than a thousand different kinds of stomachs, and he pointed out that it would be foolishness to treat each person in the same way he treated every other one, because their bodies could be as different as their spirits. "There are a hundred forms of health," he said, "and the man who can lift fifty pounds may be as able-bodied as a man who can lift three hundred pounds."

During the middle part of the 20th century, William H. Sheldon, professor of physiology at Harvard University, conducted an elaborate series of experiments in what he called "constitutional psychology," to demonstrate that human temperament was indeed related to human physique. Working with a base of 4,000 college students, he first classified humanity into three physical groups; next, he researched his subjects' backgrounds and lifestyles, and determined that specific behavior patterns were associated with the different types of physique, and that, while everyone possesses some attributes of all three types, it is the nature of the mixture that influences— not determines, however—a person's temperament.

As Robert S. DeRopp illustrates Sheldon's theory,

> Shakespeare's three prototypes, Falstaff, Hotspur, and Hamlet, correspond both physically and temperamentally to Sheldon's three *morphs.* . . . Falstaff is the extreme *endomorph.* He is shaped like a barrel ("this tun of a man"), typically oval in outline. Hotspur, the fiery fighter, is the extreme *mesomorph,* muscular, broad-shouldered, narrow-hipped, triangular in outline. Hamlet, the irresolute thinker, is lean and angular, linear in outline, the typical *ectomorph.* Their temperaments correspond to their physiques. Falstaff, with his passion for eating, is *viscerotonic* [stimulated by his viscera, his guts]; Hotspur, with his passion for action and risk, is *somatotonic* [stimulated by his muscles]; Hamlet, entangled in endless cerebration, is *cerebrotonic* [stimulated by his brain].

mesoderm, the middle germ layer, becomes the body's action system, responsible for its movement as well as for its basic structure. It comprises all the myofascia, including the muscles, bones, blood, and cartilage, as well as the kidneys, gonads, heart, and the dentine of the teeth.

The process of bodywork applies directly to the mesoderm, and in particular to that part of the mesoderm called the connective tissue. But since mesoderm is the bridge connecting all parts of the body with one another, bodywork can have a pronounced effect on endodermal and ectodermal systems as well. For example, bodywork cannot improve the efficiency of the lungs as a gaseous transfer mechanism, but it *can* improve the functions of the rib cage; when the functions of the rib cage improve, the efficiency of the lungs' pumping action also improves, and the efficiency of the entire respiratory system is enhanced. Again, bodywork cannot improve the efficiency of the intestines or stomach in performing their intrinsic functions, but in the course of releasing pressure in the smooth muscles of these organs and the connective tissue surrounding them, peristalsis is improved, and the entire digestive system performs with increased efficiency.

Bodywork does not affect the workings of any organs or nerves themselves, then, but it does affect the systems that contain and inform them. Because the body is an integrated unit, the better performance of any part improves the performance of all the other parts; and because the body is the hologram of the being, the enhanced performance of the body as a system is reflected in a person's overall experience of improved performance and satisfaction with life.

ECTODERM: THE BODY'S COMMUNICATIONS SYSTEM

The two principal components of the ectoderm are the skin and the nervous system. The functions of the skin are threefold: to contain the body's other parts, to protect them, and to serve as the major exchange membrane between the world inside the body and the one outside. The skin breathes, taking in oxygen and giving off carbon dioxide, and it absorbs and expels fluids in the forms of oils and waters. The skin is also the place most of us first recognize our sense of touch. Touch, however, is not a function of the skin, but rather of those nerve endings that are present in the skin as part of the body's nervous system.

The nervous system allows the body to communicate within itself from the extremities to the brain and from the brain to the extremities, and it also allows the body to communicate with the world around it. Its various functions are specialized between the brain and the spinal cord (the central nervous system) and all the rest of the body's nerves, reaching every place from which you see, hear, feel, touch, smell, or taste (the peripheral nervous system).

ENDODERM: THE LIFE SUPPORT SYSTEM

As organisms increase in complexity they become more and more concerned with acquiring specialized information from the world and taking specialized action regarding it. They become increasingly voluntary, as adults have more volition than infants, or primates have compared with insects. Voluntary control of behavior is first an ectodermal and second a mesodermal function; very little of the endoderm is ever under voluntary control.

The endoderm is composed principally of the body's major internal organs, what we speak of as the guts or the viscera. It is charged with regulating the body's internal environment and with converting those materials, energies, and information accepted into the system as a whole into something the body needs or can use in order to function and survive. As part of its conversion function the endoderm serves most of the body's internal trans-

Sheldon then went on to develop an "index of physique," a numbering scale by which a person's ecto-, meso-, and endomorphic components could be measurably compared. The index is composed of three numbers, each of which can range between one and seven, and each of which represents one of the morphs. Thus, Falstaff is a 711 on the Sheldon scale, Hotspur a 171, and Hamlet a 117. Although these sorts of extremes are far more likely to appear in literature than in life, they are no less likely than the perfectly balanced 444, which Robertson Davies describes as "the secretary of an athletic club with a rich membership and first-class catering."

Most people, Sheldon found, exhibit a dominant temperament consistent with the corresponding dominant morph, and two less-developed morphotonic components. A well-fed gourmand who likes to think hard about intellectual topics but does not like physical activity might register 625 on the Sheldon index; a very athletic woman who enjoys food but does not consider it important and does not care to think much about anything might chart 361; a lean executive who accepts playing golf at the club as one of life's responsibilities and forgets to eat lunch on occasion because he is sitting in his office planning corporate takeovers might rate a 227. Our rotund man here is an endomorph, our athlete a mesomorph, and our executive an ectomorph.

Since, as Sheldon demonstrated, people display their types in the kinds of lives they choose to lead as well as in their appearances and temperaments, we would expect a mesomorph to enjoy working with his body and should not be surprised to find mesomorphs as athletes, dancers, longshoremen, soldiers, and builders. Endomorphs, with their dominant guts, are more likely to be attuned to their feelings and emotions, and to work in slow, sedentary occupations, or where their emotions can find satisfying, gut-level expression: chefs and opera singers are classic endomorphs. Ectomorphs, who love to exercise their brains, might be expected to prevail in intellectual occupations as teachers, engineers, strategists, and planners.

By the same token, our use of language reflects the consciousness that inheres in each body's typology. The endomorph may talk in terms of consuming—"I can't stomach this" —where the mesomorph may speak in terms of action—"I can't grasp this"—and the ectomorph in terms of the mind—"I can't understand this." Given a problem, the ectomorph wants to think about it, the endomorph wants to feel into it, and the mesomorph wants to do something about it.

DeRopp points out that whatever the particular strengths may be of one's own body type, those same strengths are the barriers that may stand in the way of one's personal development. A muscular person may have to develop emotional and intellectual capacities very deliberately; an intellectual may find it difficult to eat and exercise properly; a gourmand might have to struggle against intellectual as well as physical sloth.

In addition, anyone can emphasize his or her secondary traits: a muscular, intellectual opera singer, a thin, emotional football player, and an obese, passionate general are not unheard of. As Sheldon noted, the particular strengths and tendencies of a person's physique and temperament influence, but do not determine, the shape of his or her life.

Nonetheless, in our culture the endomorphs have been maligned portation needs, carrying gases, liquids, and solids into, out of, and around within the body. The endoderm also is the physiological level from which we receive our gut feelings, which are often as important to our well-being as the information conveyed by other endodermal subsystems, such as respiration, digestion, and excretion.

The endoderm's regulatory function is accomplished through the continuous circulation of fluids inside the body both intra- and extra-cellularly; its object is *homeostasis*. Homeostasis is generally understood to be the stable, consistent, uniform state of the body's internal environment that allows our functions to be maintained normally. Although homeostasis does imply a state of constancy, it is the constancy of a balancing act, rather than that of a fixed and immobile rigidity, that amends conditions or materials whenever adaptation is necessary or desirable. It is more a process than a state. The need for homeostasis directs the body to generate acid when food is to be digested, to send heat to the surface of the skin when the cold winds blow, and to filter internal fluids to rid the body of its toxins. It keeps things changing, rather than keeping them the same, but it keeps them changing in an orderly way.

MESODERM: THE SYSTEM OF STRUCTURE AND SUPPORT

Another name for mesoderm is myofascia. *Myo* means muscle and *fascia* means binding. Mesoderm, then, is primarily composed of muscle and connective tissue. Mesoderm provides structure for the body and also allows for change in its structure, in the form of movement. Muscle is designed to accomplish the specific function of contraction: Muscle fibers shorten when triggered by nerve impulses, and it is this shortening of muscle fibers that produces body movement.

There are three types of muscle: Visceral (most organ walls), cardiac (the heart), and skeletal (the "red meat" that covers the entire body between the skeleton and the skin). Bodywork is partly concerned with skeletal muscle because that is what holds us up. But what holds us *together,* and what bodywork is most concerned with, is connective tissue. Since it both connects the body's parts and holds them together, connective tissue provides the basic framework for the body's entire structure. Like skeletal muscle, connective tissue is stress-responsive: The more demand you place on it, the more it will grow. But unlike muscle tissue, connective tissue is regenerative: When damaged or destroyed it will replace itself with new connective tissue. This is the reason bodywork can produce a lasting impact on the connective tissue no matter how badly it has been damaged.

FASCIA: THE GREAT CONTAINER

Bone, cartilage, ligaments, and tendons are the increasingly flexible forms of firm connective tissues; blood, lymph, and cerebrospinal fluid are the liquid connective tissues. In between them, neither liquid nor firm, are fascia, of which the great majority of the body's connective tissue is composed. You have seen fascia as the whitish membrane between muscle and fat on a leg of lamb, or underneath a chicken's skin. Fascia are sheaths, usually thin sheets, of connective tissue that act as envelopes for just about everything in the body. It might even be said that fascia is the great container. Fascia lines the thoracic and the abdominal cavities that contain the organs. Every organ is wrapped in fascia, every nerve is wrapped in fascia, every blood vessel is wrapped in fascia —even the bones are wrapped in a fascia called periosteum. And, of course, the muscles are wrapped in fascia.

Fascia is so pervasive that if you dipped the body in

more than anyone else, because we have such a negative fixation on the idea of being fat. Endomorphs tend to have large bellies since they have a predominance of endomorphic tissue, or guts. Even when they lose all their fat they retain a belly, which has nothing to do with their being overweight but rather with their natural body type, about which they can do nothing.

We find much more understanding of endoderm's importance in the various Oriental cultures that have recognized the guts as a principal energy center and have named it—*chi, hara, dan tien*—in accordance with the energy of the third chakra. Buddha is often portrayed with a large gut, symbolizing the great power and energy he possessed. In terms of the body's physical structure, of course, the body's center of gravity is in the guts.

some magic potion to remove everything that makes up the body except connective tissue, you would still be able to discern all the body's parts, including its organs. You would see a labyrinthine, three-dimensional framework of fascial planes dotted with holes where the bones and organs had been; but the spaces these pieces had occupied would still be surrounded by connective tissue, as they are right now. Reducing the body to its connective tissue leaves a totally interconnected fascial structure with a place for everything, even though not everything is in its place.

It is the nonfluid connective tissues that are manipulated in bodywork, in order to realign them from unnatural positions and patterns into which they have fallen or been forced. While a couple of bodywork disciplines, such as chiropractic and osteopathy, are concerned with the hard connective tissues—the bones—most others focus on the semisolid or semifluid connective elements —the ligaments, tendons, and fascia—because it is these tissues that accumulate tension.

A muscle is really a composite of muscle fiber and fascia, in that every single fiber that goes to make up what we refer to as muscle is wrapped in its own individual fascial sheath. Bundles of fascia-wrapped muscle fibers are then wrapped again in a separate fascia wrapping, and finally the whole bundle of bundles—the red meat we call muscle—is wrapped in a thicker layer of fascia called an investing fascia. When you cut through a muscle, across its length, it looks a bit like a coaxial cable, whose insulation-wrapped wires are gathered into insulation-wrapped bundles, the lot of which are wrapped in a thicker insulation. The picture is the same, although the proportions are different because fascia occupies a far narrower space between muscle fibers than insulation occupies between wires.

In its healthy state this fascia is a fine, elastic, semifluid membrane; it contains the body parts, but it also allows for their reasonably free movement. As it becomes compressed, however, it loses some of its elastic fluidity and becomes an increasingly solid, rigid membrane that prevents movement rather than allowing it, and that literally glues one part of the body to another in the manner of a weld. Fascia is capable of this sort of transformation because one of its principal elements is a protein molecule called collagen.

COLLAGEN: NOT JUST ANOTHER PRETTY FASCIA

Collagen, which has recently attracted a great deal of attention from medical scientists involved with gerontology and cosmetic surgery, has the property of being gelatinous. All gels, like the gelatin desserts we have known and loved, change their physical states as a result of relatively small changes in their energy levels. For example, when you mix a gelatin dessert on the stove, it is liquid; after a short time in the refrigerator, it becomes semisolid; if you heat it up on the stove again, it becomes liquid again; and it continues to change its state readily over a temperature range of less than 100 degrees Fahrenheit—a small change in the range of thermal energy.

Collagen exhibits the same capacity to change its state as does a gelatin dessert; but since there is no free collagen in the body, and since the body is maintained at a fairly constant temperature, collagen never becomes entirely liquid; it responds to biological, rather than to thermal, energy. When any part of the body is tense, its biological energy falls, because fluid flow is reduced in the area of those tissues. First, compression reduces the size of the space between molecules; hence, the fluid-carrying vessels become constricted. Less fluid arriving to the tissues means fewer nutrients supplied to them, and reduced nutrient intake results in diminished energy, as we can see by looking at any starving organism. Second, reduced fluid flow reduces the efficiency of waste product removal from the tissues. As a result, uric and lactic acids, as well as other wastes, remain in the compressed tissues, further reducing their efficient functioning. Third, because the areas are compressed, large mineral molecules (such as those of calcium) are more easily trapped in the tight spaces between cells than they are in uncompressed regions, reducing efficient functioning yet further.

In an area where biological energy is reduced, the fascial collagen begins to set, in much the same way that a gelatin dessert sets in the refrigerator. As the collagen sets, the fascia grows harder and less flexible. Much of the pain associated with tense musculature does not involve the muscle fibers themselves but results from increasing rigidity of the connective tissue enveloping the muscle fibers. And because connective tissue is stress-responsive, the fascia adapts to the new demand placed upon it until the state of tightened musculature becomes effectively permanent.

Fortunately, "effectively permanent" is not the same as "irrevocably permanent." If the gelatin dessert is left in the cool refrigerator, it remains semisolid. But as we observed, if thermal energy is restored to it by reheating, it liquifies again. The same thing happens regarding the infusion of biological energy through pressure and movement, to the rigidified fascial collagen: The gel unsets and becomes more elastic, and the tissues are restored to something like their original state of flexibility, permitting the fluid movement that is natural to the musculature.

At its most basic level the process of bodywork is one of permitting the reintroduction of biological energy to the rigidified collagen in the fascia and surrounding tissues through the use of pressure and manipulation. As the fascia are returned to their maximally fluid state, the body can regain its normal, flexible, elastic condition.

BODYWORK: SOME VARIETIES OF PHYSICAL EXPERIENCE

4

From all the time and money Americans have lavished on physical fitness in the past decade, it would seem that what is important about bodywork would be well established in our national thinking. But this is not the case. Our efforts at exercise are well-intentioned in that they strive to improve the functioning of certain body systems —especially our large-muscle groups and cardiovascular systems—and some of them certainly benefit some people sometimes. But frequently, physical fitness programs are more concerned with building up our armor, our images, and our self-protective attitudes than they are with providing any lasting physical value. Many programs concentrate on developing the outer musculature, for instance, which, as Don Johnson writes, "is useful for rapid defense. But its speed and strength are not as useful for more refined sensitivity, for subtler forms of movement, or for making love."[1]

Nor can the outer musculature alone—or in conjunction with the cardiovascular system—maintain the kind of balance that makes for easy living. Indeed, the speed and aggressiveness encouraged by many fitness programs stand in direct contrast to the major efforts of bodywork, which aim to reduce the muscular tensions that both hold and produce physical and psychological armor, to make immaterial the images we have learned to carry around with us, and to free us psychically and somatically from the habits of our attitudes. In short, it is by seeking to balance us, rather than tighten us, that the bodywork traditions seek to free us.

There are dozens of different kinds of bodywork, for the most part based in the common theme that people live fundamentally through their bodies, and that emotional, mental, and spiritual health depend on the organism's ability to function well through what Joel Kovel calls "the wisdom of the body and instinct."[2]

Some approaches to bodywork are concerned directly and solely with the flesh, some seek to reach the mind, and some work with the projected energy of the spirit. However a discipline seeks to bring a person to balance, its work is predicated on a plan to enable the body to express itself as well as possible according to its innate design; for while every aspect of a person expresses his or her entire being, "no words are so clear as the language of body expression once one has learned to read it."[3]

As we have observed, balance is a fluid condition rather than a static state. Therefore, after the initial bodywork process has been completed (which may entail a single session or a longer series of ten or a dozen or more), most practitioners will advise their clients to seek periodic tune-ups to keep the body's balance harmonious. In this regard, balancing the body is analogous to aligning the wheels on your car: Once the job is done your car rides smoothly for a while, but after you take a few hard curves or bash into the curb a couple of times your wheels need to be aligned again. So it is with the body, which encounters bumps and shocks and sudden stops every day.

The diverse forms of bodywork are like tributaries of varying sizes feeding a single, enormous river, but they all derive from four principal directions, which we shall call the *energetic, mechanical, psychological,* and *integrative* traditions. The traditions themselves, like the individual disciplines we have assigned to each heading, are far more complex than a brief overview can hope to convey; but at least such an overview, with a cursory description of a few representative forms of bodywork, will identify some features that make all these different schools of thought valuable in their own ways.

THE ENERGETIC TRADITION

The energetic is probably the oldest of the four bodywork traditions because, particularly in its diffuse forms, it is closest to the primitive rites of religion and magic, to myth, and to the notion that human energy is related to and can be affected by divine, cosmic, or universal energy. At its least systematic this tradition encompasses the simple wish that the greater energy will flow through the hands of a person especially attuned to it—a healer—to make another person's ailing body well. With techniques that actually appear to vary very little from one culture to another, this tradition takes in faith healing, psychic healing, laying on hands, calling up spirits, and varieties of shamanism.[4]

The energetic tradition appears in some form in most mystic religions, has close modern ties with transpersonal psychology, and shares its philosophical bias with what Leibnitz called "the perennial philosophy." It is concerned with the "spiritual Absolute" that Aldous Huxley thought was too awesome to be expressed logically, but found intuitively accessible under certain circumstances to most people's direct experience.[5] William James claimed that perceiving the energy of this Absolute has led people to great optimism, and to faith in "courage, hope, and trust, and a correlative contempt for doubt, fear, worry . . ." as a result of which the "blind have been made to see, the halt to walk; life-long invalids have had their health restored."[6]

The energetic traditions that appear most systematic to contemporary Westerners are those based in the Indian notion of *chakras* and in the Chinese idea of acupuncture meridians. The conceptual framework that underlies the meridians and the chakras also integrates other philosophical systems that rely for their coherence on concepts of balance, including the seasons, the elements, food groups, and patterns of human activity. These approaches are obviously not restricted to energetic modes, but unify their perspectives and practices through the appreciation and use of energy configurations.

THE CHAKRAS

The Hindu chakra system best known in the West today is that of Kundalini yoga, which was translated for Western understanding nearly sixty years ago by Charles W. Leadbeater. The chakras are seven primary energy points situated within the hollow central canal of the spine; each is a focal point for a particular type of energy associated with its proximate body part.

The more freely energy flows within and between the chakras, the healthier and more alive a person feels. Practitioners of the energetic traditions perceive physical ailments to be expressions of blocks or imbalances in the energy flow. For example, eye problems are generally associated with a blocked sixth chakra, and might also appear as a difficulty—metaphorical or literal—in perceiving; a sore throat might be understood to result from failing or refusing to speak when you have something pressing to say, or from some other difficulty in communicating. Because of the association between the

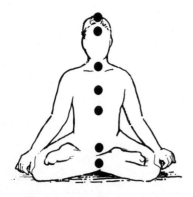

Figure 4-1. Chakras.

CHAKRA	CORRESPONDS WITH	ENERGY/FUNCTION
Seventh	Crown of head	Enlightenment
Sixth	Brow (third eye)	Insight & intuitive powers
Fifth	Throat	Communication
Fourth	Heart	Love & compassion
Third	Solar plexus (umbilicus)	Emotional & mental energy
Second	Genitals / spleen	Sex
First	Base of spine	Survival

Table 4-1

physical body and its corresponding energy body, some healers claim to be capable of curing physical as well as psychological maladies by cleaning, balancing, and adjusting the energy points the chakras are or represent.[7] One feature of most major bodywork traditions is that they release pressure along the spine, which is the physical route of the chakra system. Consequently, practitioners of the energetic tradition could justly observe that, whether by accident or design, nearly all bodywork includes energy work.

THE ACUPUNCTURE MERIDIANS

Acupuncture, an ancient Chinese healing system, assumes that the body is traversed by an intricate net of channels through which the energies of life can flow. The channels that connect major energy points are called meridians. When the flow from one meridian to the next along the channels is unimpeded, and the flowing energy is properly balanced between masculine *(yin)* and feminine *(yang)* energy, health results; physical illness, emotional distress, pain, disease, and disability signify that the energy flow is blocked or imbalanced. Stimulating the proper meridians by inserting and withdrawing extremely fine needles can affect the energy flow and set the balance right again.

Although acupuncture texts identify about one thousand different energy meridians in the human body, twelve are considered of major importance. Ten of these correspond to internal organs (bladder, gall bladder, heart, kidneys, large intestine, liver, lungs, small intestine, spleen, stomach), and two correspond to body functions (one to sex and respiration, the other to circulation). Acupuncture points along a meridian affect the related organ or function, as well as a system of organs, functions, and emotions associated with it. Energetically imbalanced kidneys, for instance, may result in lower-back pains, and may be balanced by treating the small hollow between the base of the thumb and the wrist.

THE MECHANICAL TRADITION

The mechanical tradition in bodywork is founded in the varied relationships among the body's tangible parts. Unlike people who work in the energetic tradition, those who favor body mechanics are usually concerned only with what they can touch, and do not look beyond the strictly physical. They understand the body to be for the most part an interrelated system of pulleys, levers, hinges, and plates that may become worn or misaligned because of stress and tension and, therefore, may require adjustment. Different schools within the mechanical tradition have focused on different parts of the body in their endeavors to correct imbalances. There are many discrete schools in the mechanical tradition; to give you a sense

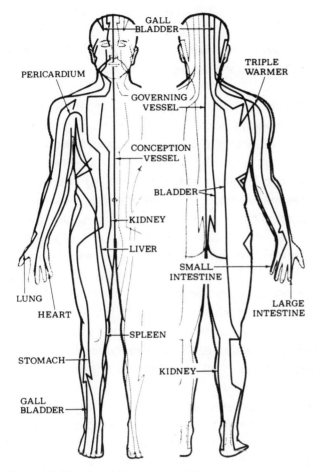

PERICARDIUM
GALL BLADDER
TRIPLE WARMER
GOVERNING VESSEL
CONCEPTION VESSEL
BLADDER
KIDNEY
LIVER
SMALL INTESTINE
LUNG
HEART
LARGE INTESTINE
SPLEEN
STOMACH
KIDNEY
GALL BLADDER

Figure 4-2. The 12 or 14 important meridians.

of their range and diversity, we will profile just a few of the better known.

ALEXANDER TECHNIQUE

Frederick Matthias Alexander was an actor in Australia at the turn of the century who found that he regularly lost his voice when he started to perform. In trying

69

to resolve this peculiar difficulty, he discovered that many problems of voice production stem not from the larynx directly but from the position in which the head and neck—and subsequently, of course, the whole body —are held.

Practicing before a mirror, Alexander found that he could regain his voice by letting his head drop down in front while letting it rise up in back; performed in a relaxed manner, without forcing, this movement allowed his neck to lengthen from the inside, whereas lifting his face, as many singers did, compressed and shortened his neck, jamming his vocal cords and causing him to lose his voice. He left the stage to teach other people to free their own bodies for the greater ease and relaxation he had found could be attained. He worked, as Alexander technique practitioners work today, more with movement than with manipulation, and such manipulation as he employed consisted in pulling the body's joints apart very slowly and gently, teaching people over the course of a couple of years to let go of the tensions they were holding.[8]

Here is an exercise you can try that will give you a feel for the Alexander technique, although it does not specifically come from the Alexander repertoire. Put your hand on your larynx, take a deep breath, and sing a few bars with some vigor. If you are like most people, you will find that your larynx rises no later than the start of your exhalation, and if this is the case, you will find that your voice becomes "tired" after you've been singing for a short while. If you continue to sing like this for several hours a day, most days, for a number of years, as professional singers do, you are likely to develop nodes on your vocal cords that will require surgery to remove, and that may damage or destroy your vocal instrument. The problem, as Alexander might have observed, is that you are concentrating on your *result:* the vocal sound. The solution is to look at the *means* by which you produce that sound, which is breathing.

Sing again, with one hand on your larynx, but this time place your other hand on your belly or chest. If your larynx rises as you exhale, either your belly, your chest, or both will expand as you inhale, and will compress your insides as you sing.

Now prepare to sing again, placing one hand on your larynx and the other on the inverted "V" below your breast where your lower ribs meet your sternum. *Allow* yourself to inhale, rather than working to do so, so that your concentration is on your diaphragm. As this muscle drops, air is sucked into your lungs without your having to *do* anything. Your belly and chest expand naturally, to contain the air. As you sing, press your hand into that "V" in your torso, and concentrate on pushing it out with your breath. You should find that your larynx does not rise as you sing, or rises less than it did before. With practice, the larynx will actually drop as you sing this way, opening the air passage around your vocal cords rather than closing it. Your voice will not tire as easily, and you are far less likely to develop vocal nodes.

TRAGER

When Milton Trager was a seventeen-year-old body-builder, acrobat, and boxer, his manager and sparring partner used to massage him after they worked out. One day they reversed roles, and a new kind of bodywork was born. Trager discovered that true body-building lay in softening and loosening hard, rigid muscles, rather than in making them tougher and tighter. He went on to cure his father's sciatica, and then he began to help polio victims learn to move again. He practiced physical therapy during World War II and in his forties became a physician. While practicing medicine in Hawaii, he would give one of his bodywork sessions per day; in 1975 he demonstrated his technique at Esalen, and soon thereafter he moved to northern California to practice and teach.

Trager had discovered that he could release tension from the joints by shaking, rocking, or gently moving each part of the body in a rhythmic way that sent ripples through the flesh like a soft sonar wave. Wherever the undulating rhythm stopped or changed, Trager identified some rigidity blocking the natural path of this movement, as if a solid island had stopped a wave's motion in water. He could then shake or manipulate the tension free from the point of the block. The more blocks are released in this fashion, the better the body is able to assume its proper, free-flowing structure and functioning.

FELDENKRAIS: FUNCTIONAL INTEGRATION

Russian-born Israeli research physicist Moshe Feldenkrais built the Van de Graaff nuclear accelerator in Paris; he was the first judo black belt in Europe and founder of the famous Jiu-Jitsu Club de France; and he worked with the electronics division in Israel's Ministry of Defense after World War II. But his interest in Gurdjieff and the Alexander technique led him to explore the human body and to discover that each individual displays a unique set of involuntary movements that reflect and express the characteristics that underlie his or her personality.

Studying and working with people in what he called Functional Integration and Awareness Through Movement, Feldenkrais found that the only permanent part of most behavior patterns is the belief that they are permanent. Therefore, he developed a bodywork system whose primary aim is to reprogram the nervous system through movement, augmented by physical pressure and manipulation. The system works in part by expanding a client's alertness to his own sensory feelings and actions, so that he can choose, at a somatic level, to reorganize the way in which his body functions. Feldenkrais has pointed out that people get into habit patterns such as turning their eyes in the same direction they turn their heads, with the result that movement of the eye itself is reduced. Whereas the eye is capable of pointing, say, 80 degrees off center, a person's habit of swinging his head to direct his eyes toward the object of their focus by, say, 50 degrees results in a habit-pattern forming that prevents the eye from moving in its socket more than, say, 30 degrees off center.

According to Feldenkrais, it is possible to re-educate the body so that, in our example, a person might turn his eyes to the left while turning his head to the right, eventually recapturing a great deal of his previously lost movement potential. These sorts of exercises, which start to release established mechanical connections from their patterns within the nervous system, result in freer movement of the entire body.

In his book *Body and Mature Behavior,*[9] Feldenkrais expands his basically mechanical theory by proposing that negative emotions produce greater tension in the body's flexor muscles (muscles that bend parts of the body) than they do in the extensors (muscles that straighten parts of the body). As a result, the muscular tightness of undischarged anger, sorrow, and fear remain locked in the body tissues themselves, compressing those muscles that become rigid when we suppress our emotions.

CHIROPRACTIC AND OSTEOPATHY

Generally better known than Alexander, Trager, or Feldenkrais are the practices of chiropractic and osteopathy. Chiropractic is a centuries-old healing practice that aims to realign bones whose misalignment is creating pressure on nerve impulses, causing their malfunction and pain.

In 1910, Daniel David Palmer first enunciated the principles of chiropractic in his book, *The Science and Art and Philosophy of Chiropractic.* Palmer had been a student of magnetic and other alternative healing methods when, in 1895, he tried repositioning a deaf man's spine and found that the man's hearing improved. After years of study Palmer concluded that nerves become irritated and cause disease when the bones through which they pass—particularly those of the spine, and most especially the atlas, or first vertebra, at the base of the neck—are displaced. Today, Palmer's thesis has been somewhat modified: Most chiropractors believe that the tissues of the body are affected by impulses emanating from the nerves, and that pain and disease are consequences of malfunctions in these impulses, such as those caused by displacement of the vertebrae.

When you look at a skeleton you can see holes between the vertebrae of the spine: The top of each hole is at the bottom of one vertebra and the bottom of the hole is at the top of the next vertebra down. Nerves pass through these holes. A basic tenet of chiropractic is that when two vertebrae are misaligned the shape of the hole they share is changed, distorting the nerve. Because some nerves follow elaborate paths through the body, the connection between a pain in the lower right leg and a pinched nerve somewhere along the upper spine may not be apparent; but when the nerve is pinched in this fashion it can both cause pain and affect the functioning of those parts of the body with which it communicates. When a person presents a complaint to the chiropractor, the practitioner traces the nerve back to the relevant vertebra, adjusts the vertebra by pressing or twisting the spine, and thereby releases the problem condition.

In recent years many chiropractors realized that they

could adjust people's spines better if the soft tissues that hold the bones together were relaxed rather than tense. As a result, a variety of mechanical muscle relaxers have been introduced to chiropractic, such as diathermy (the use of high-frequency electric currents to generate heat in the body) and ultrasound (passing sound above the audible frequency through the body to create heat), and numerous chiropractors have taken training in acupressure technique, which is deep-pressure massage based on the acupuncture points. Their explorations have led to several new mechanical disciplines and confused the common definition of chiropractic; but the practice is still based in the manipulation of bones.

Osteopathy was founded in the 19th century by a physician named Andrew Still. Still became interested in the relationship between structure and function in the human body and wrote in 1869 that the connective tissues are at the root of all disease. Like chiropractic, but in a broader fashion, osteopathy is based in the manipulation of bones. Whereas chiropractic is concerned primarily with the spine, osteopathy is concerned with all the bones and joints. In practical terms this means that while a chiropractor would be unlikely to treat, say, a club foot, an osteopath might well attempt to manipulate the club foot's bones and joints into a more useful arrangement of parts, alleviating the condition to some degree.

ROLFING

Ida Rolf, founder of Rolfing, was familiar with osteopathy. Although she was not a practitioner, she borrowed some of that discipline's techniques in the course of developing her own system of bodywork. One of the features that distinguishes Rolf's system of structural integration from virtually every other practice in the mechanical tradition, however, is that she sought a unifying ele-

There is no psychology: there is only physiology.
—Ida Rolf

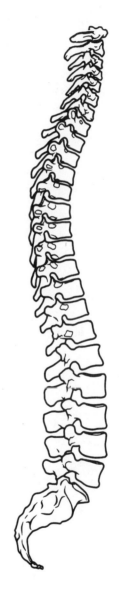

Figure 4-3. The human vertebral column.

ment for her work in the body itself. If the chiropractor would not deal with a club foot, and if the osteopath would deal with it as an isolated problem, Rolf looked for the connection between the misshapen part and the rest of the body.

Rolf found her unifying element in the relationship between the body and gravity. She sought to release blocks held in the body tissues, but recognizing that the body exists in a specific sort of physical environment that implies identifiable kinds of stress on its structure, she also worked to realign the body in a way that decreased its structural tension.

Ida Rolf perceived correlations between the body and mind as well, although she is little known for these outside the world of professional somatologists. Her explication of what we might call the "neurotic body" is quite lucid.

> An individual experiencing temporary grief, fear, or anger, all too often carries his body in an attitude which the world recognizes as the outward manifestation of that particular emotion. If he persists in this dramatization or constantly re-establishes it, thus forming what is ordinarily referred to as a "habit pattern," the muscular arrangement becomes set. Materially speaking, some muscles shorten and thicken, others are invaded by connective tissue, still others become immobilized by consolidation of the tissues involved. Once this has happened, the physical attitude is invariable; it is involuntary; it can no longer be changed basically by taking thought or even by mental suggestion. Such setting of a physical response also establishes an emotional pattern. Since it is not possible to establish a free flow through the physical flesh, the subjective emotional tone becomes progressively more limited and tends to remain in a restricted, closely defined area. Now what the individual feels is no longer an emotion, a response to an immediate situation, henceforth he lives, moves, and has his being in an attitude.[10]

THE PSYCHOLOGICAL TRADITION

Although a person's psyche can be affected through his body, as Ida Rolf clearly was aware, the psychological tradition in bodywork is not so much concerned with the health and functioning of the body itself as it is with the healthy functioning of the mind. According to this tradition, the mind can be reached *through* the body, by removing psychological blocks that manifest themselves in the living flesh. The psychological tradition in bodywork is largely founded in and promulgated by the work of two psychoanalytically trained physicians, Wilhelm Reich and Alexander Lowen.

WILHELM REICH

Reich, who was a prominent member of Freud's inner circle in Vienna, was the first Westerner to concentrate attention on the relationship between body tension, or rigidity, and psychological limitations on a person's well-being. In the therapy he developed, a person lies on a table and breathes in specific fashions dictated by the therapist, who monitors observable reactions in the client's body indicating blocks in her energy flow. Reich discovered, for example, that such blocks could be detected by the way in which skin temperature or color sometimes changes on only one side of an apparently arbitrary line on the body when a person breathes, while the skin remains unaffected on the other side of that line. Reich saw that these blocks could be released directly by physical manipulation so that color or temperature remained even across the entire body. He felt that this work, when accompanied by psychoanalysis, enhanced therapy. As Lowen later reflected, "The use of physical pressure facilitated the breakthrough of feeling and the corresponding recovery of memories. And it served to speed up the therapeutic process."[11]

In exploring what he called "the dark and difficult problems of the relationship between psyche and soma,"[12] Reich particularly felt that the touchstone of emotional difficulties was sexual experience; that a free mind in a free body would be expressed in a total body orgasm—not merely a genital one—whose regular occurrence was both essential to an individual's mental and physical health and was also impossible as long as the body was blocked anywhere.

Indeed, Reich felt that psychological tensions *could not* exist without physical parallels, nor could psychological problems be alleviated without correcting those of the body as well, because "tension and relaxation are biophysical conditions."[13] He realized that muscular and psychic rigidities were not just related but united, and that the "relaxed quality of a person's musculature accompanies flowing psychic agility."[14] Reich therefore concluded that

> a positive, affirmative attitude in life is possible only when the organism functions as a totality, when the plasmatic excitations [the blood and other fluids coursing through the body], together with the emotions pertaining to them, can pass through all the organs and tissues without obstruction, when, in short, the expressive movements of the plasm are capable of flowing freely.
>
> As soon as even one single armor block limits this function, the expressive movement of affirmation is disturbed.[15]

ALEXANDER LOWEN: BIOENERGETICS

Alexander Lowen was Reich's client, student, and colleague, and, like Reich, a physician and psychiatrist. He defined the psychological tradition in bodywork with great clarity. Throughout its development, he said,

> psychoanalysis has never been able to dissociate itself from the physical manifestations of emotional conflicts. Yet with respect to the physical function

of the organism the psychoanalytic attitude has been to approach it from its psychic reflection. One can proceed in the reverse direction with greater effectiveness; that is, from the physical problem to its psychic representation.[16]

Lowen claims that his approach, called bioenergetics—a term he borrowed from Reich, although he uses it quite differently[17]—is distinct from Reich's techniques and theories. Lowen has his clients stand up and move about the therapy room in an endeavor to make them aware of their rigidities, whereas Reich kneaded, prodded, and pounded his prone patients to break up their rigid blocks. Lowen also teaches his clients something about moving as their bodies were designed to move, rather than as their learned movement patterns dictate:

> I place a heavy folded blanket or mat on the floor and ask my patient to stand in front of it, so that when he falls, he will land on the blanket. . . .
> He is then asked to put all his weight on one leg, bending that knee fully. The other foot touches the floor lightly and is used only for balance. The directions are very simple. The person is to stand in that position until he falls, but he is not to let himself fall. Letting one's self down consciously is not falling since the person controls the descent. To be effective, the fall should have an involuntary quality. If the mind is set on holding the position, then the fall will represent the release of the body from conscious control. . . .
> In one respect this exercise resembles a Zen koan in that the ego or will is challenged, yet rendered powerless. One cannot stay in this position indefinitely yet one is obliged to use his will not to let himself fall. In the end, the will must yield, not by a voluntary act but by the superior force of nature, in this case gravity. One learns that giving in to the superior forces of nature does not have to have a destructive effect and that one does not have to use his will constantly to fight these forces. Whatever its origin, every holding pattern represents in the present the unconscious use of the will against the natural forces of life.[18]

At the same time, there are numerous similarities between these two psychological bodywork disciplines. For Lowen, as for Reich, the important feature of any human activity is whether it builds up or releases energy from the individual's biosystem; and for Lowen, as for Reich, the primary mode of energy discharge is sexual. Complete orgasm was the *sine qua non* of health for Reich,[19] who also felt complete orgasm was only possible in heterosexual intercourse. For Lowen the sexual act is the critical phenomenon of energy discharge;[20] to withhold energy in or from the sex act results in neuroses of the mind, which have direct correlatives in what we have called neuroses of the body. To treat the body, then, is to treat the mind; and the analytic portion of bioenergetics resembles the analytic portion of Reichian and other psychologically oriented therapies, with therapist and client together examining ways in which the newly recognized energy can be understood, released, integrated, and turned to productive pursuits.

THE INTEGRATIVE TRADITION

At the risk of greatly oversimplifying a complex collection of overlapping disciplines, philosophies, and approaches to bodywork, in general it might be said that practices within the energetic tradition attempt to treat underlying causes in order to clear up symptoms; that those in the mechanical tradition treat the symptom for itself; and that in the psychological tradition symptoms are addressed in order to get at whatever problems underlie them.

While the energetic, mechanical, and psychological traditions each seek to return the body to balance by emphasizing one approach over all others, there are also practices that are integrative to begin with. Such practices are likely to devote some attention to balancing the body

mechanics, some to exploring the psychological connections between physical misalignment and emotional or
mental distress, and some to balancing the body's energy
fields. In addition, many include meditative exercises that
lead to peace of mind. Most of the meditative forms of
bodywork start from the premise that life is flowing, fluid,
and constantly changing, and most of these are based in,
or are themselves, Eastern disciplines such as yoga and
the martial arts.

The word *yoga* is derived from the Sanskrit root *yuj,*
meaning to bind, attach, join, and yoke, to direct and
concentrate one's attention. Often in the practice of yoga
a kind of psychic meditation is combined with physical
exercises that realign the body, so that the integration of
body, mind, and spirit takes place all in a single, balanced
act. Yoga postures, called *asanas,* are designed to affect
particular organs and muscles, yet it takes very little practice to discover that they affect a person's thoughts, feelings, and attitudes as well.

There are many forms of martial arts practiced in the
East, ranging from the graceful dances of Ai Ki Do to the
dramatic assertions of Tae Kwan Do. Those that have
become popular in the West over the past couple of
decades usually do not involve weapons and teach people to rely on their own bodies for purposes of self-
defense. All of them devote considerable attention to
balancing the practitioner's psychological, physical, and
energetic elements, because until the body is balanced
both at rest and in motion, a person cannot truly recognize how her outer and inner environments reflect one
another, and how she is the embodiment of both, as well
as the fulcrum around which they hover. By maintaining
balance and poise we learn how the energy around us
affects our own balance, and in so doing learn to direct
our energy so that it can influence our surroundings.

One significant difference between yoga and the

martial arts and all the other bodywork disciplines we have discussed in this book is that they require long years of practice to produce results. You cannot go for a series of ten Judo classes and expect your body's alignment to be transformed: You must repeat the disciplined meditations, poses, and exercises until you have trained yourself to an entirely new way of being in the world; it is this new way of living that entails the balance and harmony with which all bodywork traditions are concerned.

The very fact of being balanced obviates many psychological issues and allows others to appear in such a new light that they cease to be experienced as problems. To be integrated, as we observed early in this book, is to be complete and whole, and it is exactly the end of completeness and wholeness that the integrative bodywork traditions serve.

In one sense, the integrative tradition is concerned with the concept of heaven. Many religious traditions teach that the state of bliss and ecstasy is something to be experienced "later," in the special place of the afterlife. But the integrative traditions implicitly propose to bring heaven down to Earth, allowing participants to experience its grace right here, right now. Heaven ceases to be seen as something *extra*ordinary to life; instead it becomes something to be experienced in the course of *ordinary* life.

ENVISIONING HELLERWORK

The structural bodywork developed by Joseph Heller, like the practice of yoga, is based in the experience of the body as the hologram of the being. Like the martial arts, it is designed to integrate the principles of the mechanical, psychological, and energetic traditions *as they are lived:* not in exercises or in a teaching or bodywork session, but in the practical tasks and functions of daily life.

Joseph Heller studied with Ida Rolf, was a Rolfer for

six years, and was the first president of the Rolf Institute. Although he patterned his approach to a bodywork series on the ten-session Rolfing program, he realized that restructuring the body is often not enough to accomplish the long-term, permanent change bodywork envisions. Habit leads even the restructured body back toward its familiar patterns—and to some of its familiar problems. As Ken Dychtwald has written, "the greatest changes in the physical body occur when there are corresponding changes in awareness and attitude."[21] In order to counteract the human tendency to drift back to the way things used to be, Hellerwork incorporates movement education for newly realigned bodies, teaching people to sit, stand, bend, walk, and balance themselves in keeping with their newly balanced structures.

The difference between Hellerwork and most other Western bodywork traditions is roughly analogous to the difference between the preventive, holistic Western medicine of recent years and the curative, symptomatological Western medicine of the early 20th century: Rather than treating a condition and sending his client back to her old ways of living, the Hellerwork practitioner seeks a fundamental change in the condition of his client's life. In this approach Hellerwork may be regarded as psychosomatic education.

Hellerwork is concerned with the way in which the body expresses a person's psychology. As Reich, Lowen, Feldenkrais, and others would recognize, people are *always* perfectly self-expressive through their bodies, both consciously and unconsciously, advertising their attitudes and beliefs in their postures and movements. For instance, the person walking around with slumped shoulders is likely to be using his body to say he feels burdened. If the condition is temporary, the slumped shoulders may also be temporary; but if the condition is chronic, as Ida Rolf knew, it ceases to be volitional, and the person's whole life actually comes to feel like a bur-

One morning . . . Ida Rolf clumped into her living room at Big Sur where about twenty of us were assembled. "Word's going around Esalen that Ida Rolf thinks the body is all there is. Well, I want it known that I think there's more than the body, but the body is all you can get your hands on."
—Don Johnson, *The Protean Body*

den to him. During Hellerwork a client is encouraged to explore the feelings bodywork raises, to discover where and when he began to adopt the mental attitudes and beliefs that led to his self-presentation. Without such an exploration, the habit of the physical attitude can dominate even some of the restructuring bodywork can accomplish.

If a Hellerwork practitioner is working on a client's shoulders, for example, and the client discovers she is feeling anger, the practitioner and client may talk a bit about the feelings and their origin as those feelings are reflected in her body. Perhaps the client discovers she has opened up a trove of anger stored from events in the past, whose expression she has restrained. It is, of course, beneficial for her to experience the release of that anger as she might do in psychotherapy; but in bodywork it is more beneficial for her to realize that by holding back the experience of anger she has also prevented herself from having some of aggression's positive results—such as reaching out for those things that are supportive and nourishing and taking care of herself.

Hellerwork assists such a person to see aggression in a balanced way: not simply as anger or hostility that is to be feared and held back, but as a continuum of expression in an outward orientation called "reaching" that ranges from reaching *against* something (pushing it away) to reaching *for* something (drawing it closer). Hellerwork points out that one can have aggression in love as well as in anger, and that if one holds back the experience of anger, one will automatically hold back (or hold oneself back from) the experience of love at the same time.

As Hellerwork highlights psychological issues and patterns embodied by the physical structure, it also explores energy, starting with gravity and including the sense of connection people can discover between themselves and the universe beyond them. In this sense it is a practice of inclusion, rather than exclusion.

84

Hellerwork combines deep-tissue bodywork with movement awareness. The sessions develop thematically, building upon one another, each one addressing a specific theme representing a major polarity in human life, such as up/down, right/left, back/front, and masculine/feminine. In examining independence, for instance, Hellerwork clarifies the dependence/independence polarity. The seventh Hellerwork session, which involves the head, is concerned with reason and passion, as well as finding the balance between them. In each session the practitioner releases habitual mechanical, psychological, and energetic patterns that have restricted the body's alignment. Corresponding movement work integrates the structural change into normal life activities, enhancing the client's flexibility, grace, vitality, ease of movement, and—hence—sense of well-being.

Hellerwork is based on principles of alignment, gravity, balance, and fluidity. Stressful physical patterns and habits are not seen as "bad" things to be eliminated, but as responses that may once have been appropriate to a situation that no longer exists. Release of the rigidified musculature is, itself, a teaching aid through which the practitioner enables the client to see what her body has done in the past, what effect its doing so has had in the present, and what choice she has about realigning her relationship with her own mechanical, psychological, and energetic components, as well as with those of other people.

Movement is the context of Hellerwork, in that Hellerwork is primarily concerned with affecting the range and quality of movement by working on the movement of the structure, rather than on the structure itself.

When you take your car to the mechanic for a tune-up, he may get involved with the spark plugs and fan belts and fuel pump because these aspects of the car interest him. As a driver, on the other hand, you may have no interest at all in mechanics. You just want your car to start when you turn on the ignition, and when you drive you want the car to be responsive to your commands.

Like the automobile mechanic, the Hellerwork practitioner becomes involved with the mechanics of the body's structure, whereas most of her clients are primarily concerned with how well it moves and functions in day-to-day activities.

Hellerwork, then, is a "moving experience" because part of the work is directed to restoring to the client an increased range of motility, by educating him to those movements that are most efficient and effective for his unique structure, in order to enable him to maintain a state of balance and ease.

Lao Tzu said that if you give a hungry man a fish you feed him for a day, but if you teach him how to fish you feed him for a lifetime. Both actions are helpful, but they constitute help of entirely different orders. In the long run, it is only help of the second kind that can return a person to himself; but until the short-term need is met, few people can attend to their long-term growth. Hellerwork strives to provide both kinds of help, filling the immediate needs of the client in order to reach the state where he can help himself. And this is the final integrative aspect of Hellerwork—that it is a practice of reaching the mind and spirit as well as the body, which is the hologram of the entire being.

In the remainder of this book we will explore the way the Hellerwork series balances, aligns, and integrates the body, step by step. Each session will be addressed in a separate chapter, except where combining themes will make understanding Hellerwork's perspective easier, such as in the single chapter on balancing masculine and feminine energies. There are many different kinds of bodywork, each effective in its own way. By examining this one system in detail, we will provide a model for the advantages of *any* bodywork.

PART TWO:
BODY OF KNOWLEDGE

INTRODUCTION

5

HELLERWORK AND THE BODY OF KNOWLEDGE

Most Americans do not work very hard physically. We drive or ride almost everywhere we go, and when we arrive we mostly sit. Such exercise as we get is usually recreational and would not be considered strenuous by any normally functioning human being who had lived anywhere on Earth until the second half of the 20th century. The question, though, is not whether we are fortunate, lazy, or self-indulgent; rather, it is, Why are so many of us so very tired at the end of our easy days?

The answer is that, although we spend little time in activities that make physical demands on us, we expend a lot of physical effort unnecessarily. We live as if we believe life is hard, as if we must struggle, as if we have to exert vast effort to be what we want, do what we want, and have what we want.

We translate this attitude into the smallest and most common of our acts. We grip our pencils so hard when we write that our hands ache. We clench our thighs, buttocks, and abdomens so tightly when we sit we develop hemorrhoids. We hold our backs so rigidly out of balance that 75 million Americans—nearly half this country's adult population—have back pain serious enough to take to physicians, chiropractors, or bodyworkers. We hold onto the steering wheels of our cars as if wild vehicles would stampede down the highways of the land were we ever to relax, while our shoulders and necks quiver with the effort, and tension pain in our heads, eyes, and jaws sends us reeling for aspirin, Valium, and gin. It is not the work we do on our jobs so much as the work our ingrained habits demand that saps our strength and results in our feeling far more fatigued than our apparent levels of activity would seem to warrant.

The experience of life lived as if it is hard translates itself into stress and rigidity in our bodies—literal hardenings of the tissues, which cause us pain, discomfort, and dis-ease. A great deal of what takes place in the course of Hellerwork involves removing this accumulated rigidity from the body, allowing the tissues to return to their original, fluid states. This task is accomplished in three ways: through deep-tissue bodywork on a massage table; in movement education that teaches clients more efficient ways of using their bodies than they have known before; and in dialogues with the practitioner that allow clients to examine the attitudes, feelings, thoughts, and beliefs that have to some degree shaped their bodies and made them what they are today.

Deep-tissue bodywork reduces the accumulated tension and rigidity stored in the body and reorganizes the structures of the body by working with the connective tissue known as *fascia,* a term that means "binding" in Latin. As we discussed earlier, connective tissues literally hold the various parts of the body together, wrapping the body's components, including muscles, nerves, organs, blood vessels, and bones. These wrappings are all interconnected so that the whole body can be seen as something like a three-dimensional maze of interwoven fascial layers.

90

In its natural state, fascia is made up of thin, lubricated, elastic sheets that facilitate the movements of the body's different parts. For instance, it allows one muscle to slide over an adjoining muscle when you sit down or turn your head. As tension and rigidity accumulate, however, the fascia degenerates. It becomes dry, loses its elasticity, and acquires the consistency of glue. The degenerating layers of fascia literally glue themselves to other layers of fascia, impeding rather than facilitating muscle movement. Then, when you move one muscle you actually have to drag several others along. As a result, your range of movement deteriorates and becomes painful, and a general rigidity sets into the body that we have come to associate with the aging process.

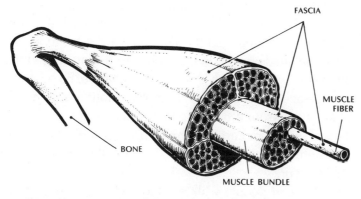

FASCIA

MUSCLE FIBER

BONE

MUSCLE BUNDLE

Figure 5-1. Fascia wraps all the muscles, muscle bundles, and muscle fibers in the body, as well as the bones, organs, and nerves.

On the table, the Hellerwork practitioner applies pressure to the sheets of tense fascia, loosening them, separating them where they have become stuck, and restoring their fluidity, elasticity, and free movement. The practitioner also works with the client to reintegrate parts of the body, improving their alignment with each other and with gravity.

Because our bodies are held together by connective tissue, they do not simply topple over when they are out of alignment, despite gravity's force. But when our bodies are twisted and out of balance, gravity pulls us farther off center—in the direction toward which we are inclined—and places enormous, unnatural stress on the muscles and fascia of the misaligned body, demanding that we exert great physical energy simply to hold ourselves upright.

It is fairly simple to demonstrate that the more aligned a body is with gravity, the less it suffers stress. Take the head and neck, for instance: The upright human structure is designed so that the head can sit directly on top of a vertical neck, which can sit directly on top of the shoulders. In this position the body can support the head with little stress or effort. But when the neck tilts forward, the head loses its support and is inclined to roll off in the direction of the tilt. In response to the pressure of this inclination, the muscles in the back of the neck that are attached to the back of the skull become tense trying to keep the head upright. Because the discomfort caused by such stress and tension is structural in nature, no amount of massage or rubbing or mentholated lotion or infrared heat or ultrasound can possibly eliminate the problem. Any of these aids can ease the pain temporarily, but once the sufferer resumes normal activities, the tension and stress recur.

A lot of people walk around with their heads and necks in front of their torsos, so it is no surprise that tension in the muscles of the head and the back of the neck is among the most frequent complaints of people who seek bodywork. Structurally, it is precisely this head and neck tension that accounts for three common ailments seen by bodyworkers: (1) tension headaches, which result from tension spreading forward to the temples and forehead; (2) vision problems, which may be caused or exacerbated by tension spreading forward along the band of connective tissue that encompasses the eyes; and (3) temporo-mandibular joint (TMJ) dysfunction, which is a disorder of the jaw hinge immediately below the temples. (You can feel the TMJ at work right in front of your ears if you open and close your mouth.) Tension that spreads forward from the back of the neck is a significant factor contributing to TMJ disorders, which are an increasingly common problem for dentistry.

Since the body is an integrated system, a misalignment anywhere will produce a corresponding misalignment elsewhere. For this reason, Hellerwork proceeds as an interrelated series of eleven ninety-minute sessions, rather than as isolated pieces of work, balancing not only the head, neck, and shoulders, but the entire physical organism. Yet, because we humans are creatures of habit, simply reducing tension and realigning structure are not enough to effect a completely satisfactory physical change. What is needed is a process of re-education. The bodywork client has to learn to use his body effectively, not in the esoteric poses of yoga or the exotic physical disciplines of the martial arts, valuable as those can be, but in the most basic, everyday motions such as standing up, sitting down, walking, and bending over to pick things up. Movement education, like all the other aspects of Hellerwork, is about everyday life. The most common thing we all do when awake is sit. Since you have been sitting virtually all your life, you know pretty well how to do it. You might notice how you are sitting in your chair right now, without trying to change your posture. You will probably find that you are sitting in such a way that your pelvis, your hip area, is tilted back. (If you are unsure where the line of your pelvis is, it is approximately the same as the beltline of your clothing. If your beltline is tilted so that the back is lower than the front, your pelvis is also tilted that way.) If you imagine your pelvis in its

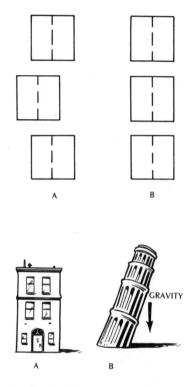

Figure 5-2. When we are well and properly aligned, gravity supports us as it supports a house that is standing up. (A) When we fall out of alignment, gravity pulls us down like the Leaning Tower of Pisa. (B)

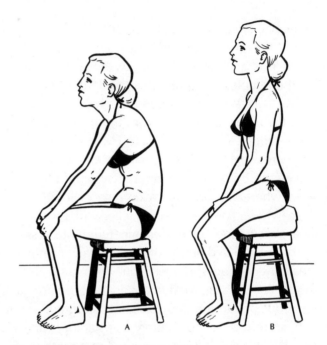

Figure 5-3. Slouching (A) and sitting (B).

present position as a bowl holding water, you probably recognize that the water should be spilling over the rim at your back.

Now, exaggerate that backward pelvic tilt and let your chest settle down on top of your pelvis. The attitude you're aiming for is what is known as *slouching.* Slouching is a very common way of sitting, much encouraged by the design of our furniture, which leads us to sit with our knees higher than our hip joints and our pelvises thrust back. As you slouch, you probably have noticed that your shoulders are rounded and your shoulders, neck, and head are slumping forward. Also notice what is happening to your rib cage, and try taking a deep breath without changing your position. As you can feel, breathing takes a lot of effort in a misaligned body.

Now, sit so that your pelvis is reasonably horizontal: You may have to move your feet under your chair and not rest against its back in order to level out. Once your pelvis is straight, let your chest rest in what is now a normal position and take another deep breath. You will notice that the second position supports your rib cage far better than the first, and that breathing is much easier. A Hellerwork practitioner could free your chest from every kind of tension, realign it in perfect accord with gravity, and make it possible for you to breathe quite freely, but all his work and all your new-found ability would be wasted if you then continued to sit in a slouch, which inhibits the kind of free movement bodywork helps you to develop.

Once a part of the body has been realigned in Hellerwork, the practitioner teaches the client to move in ways that support the natural design functions of that body part without expending energy unnecessarily, and that allow for maximum comfort with minimum distress. This phase of movement education is intended to educate people to make optimum use of their bodies.

The third feature of Hellerwork concerns people's emotions, attitudes, thoughts, and beliefs, and it works in concert with the first two parts. Recall the type of person we discussed a few pages ago, whose head and neck are thrust forward and whose shoulders are slumped. Her whole attitude expresses the feeling that life is a burden. If that attitude is situational (for instance, if the rent is overdue, she has just broken up with her boyfriend, her best suit was ruined at the cleaners, and she walks out of her home late for work only to find her car has been towed), it presents no significant problem for her physical well-being; but if it is chronic, and if it predominates in her life, no amount of realignment and movement education will take hold. She may leave her Hellerwork sessions standing upright and moving freely, but sooner or later she will feel depressed and burdened by life, she will express her feelings by slumping her shoulders, and her

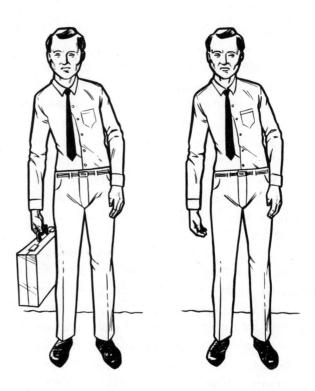

Figure 5-4. The simplest sorts of everyday activities can throw our bodies out of alignment, and their effects may stay with us even when the original cause seems to be gone. Our misalignments become chronic as we fight with gravity to maintain our balance, creating whole new misalignments over which we fight with gravity yet more. Unless we can return to a condition and position of alignment we are destined to fight a losing battle, being dragged down all the way by just that force —gravity—that could help us remain upright if we could only stop the struggle.

own internal patterns will reshape her body to conform with her fundamental attitude.

In the course of the Hellerwork series, the practitioner and client hold an ongoing dialogue, part of whose purpose is to elicit those of the client's emotions and attitudes that pertain to the part of the body under consideration in each session. The attitudes, thoughts, beliefs, and emotions that in general have emerged as most common constitute the themes of the eleven Hellerwork sessions: Inspiration; Understanding (or, Standing on Your Own Two Feet); Reaching Out; Control and Surrender; Gut Feelings (or, Letting It All Hang Out); Holding Back; Losing Your Head; Feminine Energy; Masculine Energy; Integration; and Coming Out (or, Empowerment). The organization of the first ten sessions reflects the ten-session bodywork sequence originally developed by Ida Rolf.

The first three of the eleven sessions concern the superficial, or extrinsic, musculature of the body, called the *sleeve*. The sleeve is composed of large muscles connecting the limbs to the trunk, with which we move, walk, and pick things up. The fourth through the seventh sessions are devoted to the central, intrinsic core of the body consisting of the spine, vertebrae, and the little muscles that connect the vertebrae to the ribs and to each other, as well as connect the spine to the pelvis. These structures are concerned first with support and second with fine movement. The last four sessions concentrate on integrating core and sleeve, and on the emanation of body movement from deep rather than from superficial issues, such as control and surrender, the use and restraint of power, and the responses of the gut.

The sessions proceed by separating the body into functional—not necessarily anatomical—systems in a coherent, logical pattern; but they also emphasize relations among those systems so that the body itself can be experienced as a component of the integrated unit that is the whole person. The themes of the Hellerwork sessions recapitulate the individual human development, both physically and psychologically. The first three sessions, for instance, are themes of early childhood, relating to breathing, standing by yourself, and reaching out for what you need. The next four sessions concentrate on the concerns of adolescence: finding a personal identity, discovering sexuality and true autonomy, and freeing yourself from childhood restraints along the way to achieving both physical and societal maturity. The remaining sessions are concerned with issues of adulthood: establishing balance and equanimity within the scope of your personal forces, integrating what you have learned in the course of growing up, and expressing yourself fully and as an equal in the world of adults.

Each of the Hellerwork themes will be considered in some depth in the ensuing chapters of this book, as we explore the ways each one of us integrates body, mind, and spirit based in these eleven areas.

In these chapters we will examine the body as a channel for the flow of life's energy, whatever that phrase may mean to you. Some people think of life energy in a spiritual way, as the Indian *prana* or the Chinese *chi* or some other sort of motive force. Other people prefer to see it intellectually or emotionally as a reasonable or passionate set of thoughts, feelings, or beliefs; still others understand the energy in biological terms, as the nutrients that feed the flesh. Hellerwork embraces all these approaches equally. Whatever the energy of life means to you, Hellerwork addresses it, because Hellerwork starts with the most tangible part of the human being, the body; and whatever the life force means to you, you can find it in the living body.

It is commonly believed that over time the body, this channel for the flow of life's energies, deteriorates. It is supposed to become plugged up like the rusting pipes in a house so that less and less energy can flow through it until the whole thing just clamps shut. Such a belief is related to the notion that our bodies are accidents that just happened to us: that we had nothing to do with creating them. It is also related to the idea that wherever you may be in the course of life, except for early childhood, it's all downhill from here; and to the assumption that there is nothing you can do about any of these cir-

Don St. John, a Hellerwork practitioner and former psychotherapist, has organized a developmental model for the eleven Hellerwork sessions, comparing them to Erik Erikson's Eight Stages of Man.

HELLER	ERIKSON
Inspiration	Basic trust of the infant in life, leading to hope and a drive toward self-sufficiency (infant)
Understanding, or, Standing on Your Own Two Feet	Sense of autonomy, leading to self-control and the emergence of willpower (toddler)
Reaching Out	Personal initiative, leading to a sense of purpose and direction (pre-school),
	and
	Industry, leading to self-motivation, competence at learning tasks appropriate to the society, and a resulting sense of accomplishment (school-age)
Surrender and Control	Personal identity, leading to the ability to be faithful and devoted (adolescence)
Gut Feelings, Holding Back, and Losing Your Head	Ability to be intimate with self and others, leading to affiliations and love (young adult)
Feminine Energy and Masculine Energy	Generativity, leading to the ability to be productive and to care about the larger world (middlescence)
Integration and Coming Out	Ego-integrity, leading to love of the human experience, an idea of life's order, and a spiritual sense of its purpose and inevitability (old age)

Table 5-1

cumstances or conditions: You can either resign yourself to them or you can fight them, but basically you're stuck. This collection of attitudes, particularly the last, determines what many people do for their bodies. We exercise and diet and condition ourselves at spas in a variety of ways, but all our effort is based on the premise that ours is a losing battle, an inevitable downhill slide despite our ability to scramble back up a few feet now and then.

Hellerwork is based on a different set of assumptions, the first of which is that we are responsible for our bodies. We grow and alter our bodies many times to fit our changing acts, and we grow up the way we do partly to express ourselves in particular ways. Our bodies are the tangible results of these choices and of our basic attitudes toward ourselves.

The second assumption in Hellerwork is that we do have a choice about many of the things that seem to go on in our bodies without our consent. We can change our bodies through manipulation and education, without surgery, exercises, or diets.

The third assumption is that life can be better from now on, rather than worse. Most people think of aging as an inevitable deterioration of the body that results from the passage of time. Yet we all know some fifty-year-olds who are chipper and vigorous and others who look as if they have one foot in the grave, so clearly the simple passage of time is not the culprit. What is? Genes, you may answer, or some other sort of luck or fate. But Hellerwork sees the deterioration commonly ascribed to aging as the accumulation of tension and rigidity in the body. It has been the experience of many practitioners and even more clients that when tension and rigidity are taken out of the tissues and movement is restored to them, people feel and look more vital, relaxed, and younger than they did before bodywork. This is not to say that Hellerwork can transform a sixty-year-old into a thirty-year-old, but rather that the sixty-year-old can become capable of moving like a thirty-year-old. Aging need not be accompanied by the rigidity, tension, and tissue deterioration that has traditionally been associated with it.

In terms of the mind, our society gives people two basic choices as they grow old: Either become wise or become senile. One choice is a positive option resulting from the accumulation of years. But in terms of the body we offer people only the equivalent of senility: The body can only get worse. From the perspective of Hellerwork this is simply not so. There is a physical equivalent to wisdom, which entails the ability to have energy flow through the bodily channel, improving with time so that a person's ability to experience and feel fully the joys and passions and depths of life can expand, and so that people can feel more, not less, vibrant, vital, and alive as time goes on. This is the choice of living a life of ease, balance, and integrity.

INSPIRATION

6

THE THORACIC CAVITY

During the first session of Hellerwork the practitioner may ask the client, What inspires you? Clients have answered, My family; My work; Sex; Seeing great beauty in nature; Peace; My lover; Money; God. Inspiration fills each of us according to who we are, where we are in our lives, and what we find deeply moving. What inspires us is what enables us to be connected with the wellsprings of meaning for ourselves. Inspiration opens us up, delights us, thrills us, makes us gasp, and lets us draw the wonders of living deeply into ourselves. What inspires you? What energizes you, motivates you, excites you, turns you on?

Inspiration is a word with a double meaning in English. It denotes both the physical inhalation phase of the breathing cycle and the metaphysical taking in of spirit or life force. Like the two experiences, the word's two meanings are intimately related. Freeing the body's breathing structures from patterns of muscular rigidity

All ideas rise like music from the physical.
—Guy Davenport, *Eclogues*

and tension, which is the purpose of the first Hellerwork session, simultaneously expands a person's ability to feel and express high levels of energy.

BREATH AND THE BODY

Breathing is the very first act we must all perform on our own. It is our proclamation, the single event that signifies we are alive.

In the physical act of breathing, the upper part of the torso acts as a bellows mechanism, with the rib cage, lungs, and diaphragm functioning together essentially like an air pump. At a gross level the purpose of breathing is

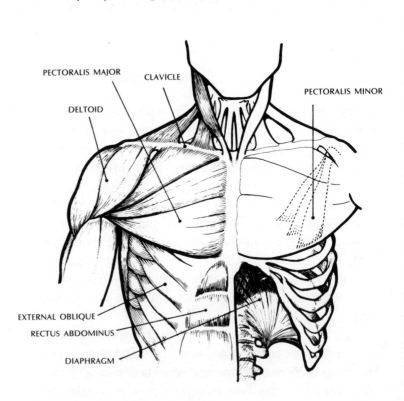

Figure 6-1. Anatomy of the rib cage.

to take in oxygen from the environment and to expel waste gases from the body. A subtler gas exchange also takes place as a result of these large breathing movements, one that fuels every one of the body's cells and triggers or initiates those energy-processing reactions we discussed earlier in this book. Breathing literally energizes —turns on—the entire body.

If you feel your own torso right now, you will find its upper portion is reinforced with ribs, while the lower section is an unreinforced muscular wall. The difference is a matter of design function: The upper, or thoracic, cavity is largely an air chamber, whereas the lower, abdominal, cavity is largely a fluid chamber. Since liquid is, for all intents and purposes, not compressible, the contents of the abdomen provide inherent support to the structure that contains them. But since air is highly compressible, the hollow upper chamber requires external support if it is not to collapse in the course of ordinary life. In addition to providing this support, the ribs are designed to expand and contract with the bellows's rhythmic inhalation and exhalation of air.

The effectiveness of our breathing can be influenced by several factors, among which the most important is the efficiency of the bellows mechanism itself: how much and how well a body fills and empties its air chamber. The difference between a person's full inhalation and full exhalation is known as the *vital capacity.* It determines the amount of oxygen that is available to the body in the bloodstream. The greater the mechanism's pumping ability, the more oxygen it can provide for the blood to pick up, and the better able it is to evacuate carbon dioxide.

The second factor influencing the gas exchange is the health of the air chamber: Damaged lung tissue cannot receive clean air as efficiently as can lung tissue that is whole. The health of the lungs' delicate membranes can be affected mechanically—by surgery, for instance,

I think asthma was one of the prices I had to pay for my sense of suffocation [in childhood] and of doing my best to keep out of trouble, just for a quiet life.
—R. D. Laing, *Wisdom, Madness, and Folly*

If you are an average adult, you are using approximately 15 pints (8000 ml) of air per minute as you sit quietly reading this book.

Wilhelm Reich thought of breathing as a four-part cycle: First, a charge of energy is built up through inhalation; second, the tension of the charge is sustained by a natural pause at the apex of the breath; third, tension is discharged through exhalation; and fourth, the body relaxes. Reich's version of the breathing cycle precisely foreshadows the four-stage sexual response cycle identified by William Masters and Virginia Johnson in their studies of human sexual response: excitement, plateau, orgasm, and resolution.

and its resulting scar tissue—but the greatest damage to human lungs occurs chemically, as a result of inhaling smoke, smog, and other noxious substances that inhibit the lungs' ability to perform their functions.

Tension affects the body's vital capacity in several ways, most directly by restricting the ability of the rib cage to expand and contract. If you have ever worn a shirt or vest or jacket that was too tight, you may remember feeling unable to take a deep breath comfortably; or if, right now, you put an ordinary belt around your chest and cinched it tightly, you would feel the same kind of constriction. When we become tense and anxious with the strains of day-to-day living, that tension often settles in the upper torso, inhibiting us from taking full, free breaths. In such circumstances our vital capacity is diminished: Our lungs are unable to take in all the oxygen our bodies require, and we feel, quite literally, less alive.

Tension in life creates tension in the body tissues, as we will see throughout the second half of this book, and tension in the tissues compresses the capillaries. As a result, the quantity of blood that can reach the cells is reduced, less oxygen reaches the cells, and less waste gas can pass out of the body in normal respiration. This is how the tension you experience sitting in rush-hour traffic lodges at the deepest cellular levels of your body. Tension also affects the cellular gas exchange in a structural way, because it thickens the fine connective tissue, the fascia, that surrounds all cell membranes. When the tissue grows rigid under stress it actually becomes a barrier to the purposeful exchange of gases.

As we mentioned earlier, one function of breathing is to provide a kind of pumping action that keeps the body's fluids in motion at all times. The major fluid-connective tissues circulate as a consequence of physical movement. The only exception is arterial blood, which is pumped independently by the heart. But the body as a whole is not a dependable pump, simply because we are not always walking or jumping or running around. When we are sitting down reading a book, for instance, or lying down asleep, our fluid systems depend for their impetus on the ever-present movement of the breath. In this regard, breathing may quite literally be understood as the body's prime mover. And as important as the breath is to the body's fluids, the body's fluidity is just as important to the breath, because the more fluid the entire body is, the more the movement prompted by the breath can spread throughout the structure. Conversely, of course, the more rigid the body is, the more restricted movement becomes and the less such movement can spread.

Imagine what would happen if you put a balloon under water, with its mouth extending above the surface, and then pumped air into the balloon. You can see that a pressure wave would move through the water away from the balloon in all directions simultaneously as the balloon inflated, and that this movement would be akin to the movement you see when you drop a pebble into a pond, although in our example movement would be visible in three dimensions rather than two. In a sense, the lungs are like two such balloons inside the water of the body. When you inflate your lungs by inspiration, a pressure wave travels out through the body fluids in all directions.

As waves that travel through water stop when they hit some solid object, and as waves travel more readily through water than they do through some thicker, more viscous liquid such as oil or sludge, so it is with pressure waves in the body: The more rigid the fluid tissues are, the less dispersed the pressure wave will be and the less far it will be able to travel—the less readily it will be able to touch extremely distant parts of the body, in other words, and the less it will be able to energize them.

If you have ever watched a baby or a sleeping cat breathe, you have seen a relatively small movement in its rib cage that seems somehow to spread throughout most of the body. These bodies are not only fluid-filled, as ours are, but unlike most adult human bodies, they express themselves freely in liquid motion. In a similar way, when a bodyworker presses on the rib cage of someone who is relaxed and at ease, it feels like pressing on a basketball: The chest gives under the fingers' light pressure and springs back immediately when the pressure is released. But pressing on the rib cage when the same person is tense and wound-up feels like pressing on a barrel: There is very little give and, consequently, very little spring in return.

If your own rib cage is tight from time to time, your life may not be affected much. But it is possible for such tightness to become a chronic part of your physical structure. Then, because the systems of your body are not as liquid as they were designed to be, the energy your breath is intended to provide becomes restricted and cannot flow freely, and rigidity starts to spread throughout the tissues.

There are three principal ways by which a person accumulates a chronic rigidity in the chest: actual physical conditions such as blows that produce broken ribs, or diseases such as emphysema or asthma; habitual misuse of the thorax from physical habits such as walking about with a puffed-up swagger or a depressed or protective hunching over; and habitual emotional restriction, particularly of the emotions we regard as negative, such as fear, anger, and sorrow. The most direct solution to the structural problems such rigidities inevitably produce is to realign the torso. This gives the body access to more oxygen. The influx of oxygen diminishes fatigue and the need for sleep by increasing the body's level of energy.

Breathing becomes easier and more rhythmical when the entire body is held erect without any conscious effort.
—Moshe Feldenkrais

108

BREATH AND ENERGY

In any kind of combustion it is the mixture of air and fuel that allows oxidation, and combustion in the body is no exception. As you can control the speed with which a log burns in your fireplace by opening or closing the flue, so the quickest way to change your energy level is to alter the amount of air you take in through breathing. You know this in your body, and adjust your air intake accordingly. When you start to run, for instance, you quickly increase your rate of respiration; when you lie down, your reduced need for energy is reflected in slower, shallower breathing and reduced air consumption.

It *is* possible to take in too much oxygen, incidentally, and oxygen poisoning can lead to death. But you will not find such a quantity of oxygen available to you in the air we breathe.

Breath is not only the body's prime mover because it keeps our fluids circulating; it is also the most important, most immediate source of energy for the human body. We tend to think of food and water in this capacity, and there is no denying that food and water energize us. However, almost any person can fast for a month with no adverse effects, and may even feel better for it; most people can go for several days without water and suffer nothing greater than discomfort. But no one can go without air for more than a few minutes without severely damaging the brain.

As an expression of our emotions and personal energies, breathing also illustrates a great deal about our attitudes toward life. One person takes life in big gulps, another hangs on to every breath for fear of running out, a third likes to puff herself up by keeping her chest expanded all the time, a fourth feels deflated and walks around with his chest sunk down toward his pelvis. When

To breathe is to feel; and conversely, to limit breathing is to limit feeling.
—Ken Dychtwald

we feel joyous, elated, or relieved we increase our energy by increasing our intake of air: We breathe deeply or we shout, laugh, or sing—which requires, in its turn, that we breathe more deeply. And when we feel sad, angry, frustrated, or resentful, we diminish our energy by diminishing our breathing: We breathe less frequently or less deeply, or we even hold our breath altogether.

We also express the feeling-state of our energies through body movement in ways that affect our breathing. For example, when we are afraid we want to run, and when we are angry we want to hit. We need not act on all our feelings, but if we ignore them we are liable to repress them, and by repressing those emotions we stuff all the tension that would properly have been involved in their expression. We stiffen our necks and clench our jaws instead of acknowledging what we want to say, or we tighten our bellies rather than recognize that our feelings have been hurt.

Many small children are taught that big boys and big girls don't cry. This is patently untrue, of course, and the statement is usually a management ploy on the part of some adult who does not want to deal with a child's tears or their cause. But the child, who wants to be thought of as a big kid and wants the adult's approval, holds back the tears. You have seen the jaws of little children quiver when they are close to crying. That quivering is a sign of tension held in those parts of the body that prevent the expression of emotion.

As with other physical holding, one occasion or two or a dozen is unlikely to damage the body. But if repression becomes a repetitive pattern, the muscles accumulate a little more tension and then a little more in addition to that, until the rib cage, chest, and diaphragm become set, and the child's torso becomes chronically tight. Then he breathes less and eventually develops a physical inability to express sadness—or even to be aware of feeling the emotion—by crying.

Laughing is as much an expression of emotion as crying—the spasmodic contractions of the breathing mechanism that release tension are often quite hard to distinguish—and though it is less common, the repression of laughter has the same implications for physical rigidity as the repression of tears. In bodywork we often find that the person who cannot let go enough to cry cannot laugh freely and deeply either. *Any* posture or repression that impairs breathing affects the entire body; it reduces a person's vital capacity and energy, and inhibits the full experience of life.

Happily, the converse is also true: Expressing oneself increases the energy available in a person's life. If you care to demonstrate this proposition for yourself, sit in a chair in a very slumped position, letting your head and upper chest fall forward until your back is arched in a C-curve. Now talk to someone else about something that truly excites you, and see how incongruent your words are with your posture and the kinesthetic feeling you have in your body. What are the reactions of the person watching and listening to your incongruous presentation? How long are you able to maintain both your depressed posture and your inflated monologue? Which do you give up first?

Because breath is the primary energizer of the body, you can increase your energy level at any time by increasing your oxygen intake, or decrease your energy level by decreasing your oxygen intake. Next time you find yourself in a boring situation where you wish you could stay awake but all you seem able to do is close your eyes and doze, the quickest way to re-energize yourself is to participate: Get involved and talk about the topic at hand. Your participation itself will increase your breathing, and you will find yourself awake again, turned on.

One function of breathing is to carry our oral communications. The passage of air through the vocal cords produces the sounds our voices make, and the physical exertion of talking increases our rate of breathing. A depressed person talks in a relative monotone and breathes slowly and shallowly, whereas a very excited person more often talks in a high pitch at great speed—breathlessly, we say. The louder and more animatedly we talk, the more breath we require. If in the beginning was the word, before that there must have been a deep inspiration: Talking makes us breathe, and we have to breathe to talk.

The importance of breath in talking makes not breathing—or breathing minimally—an effective way to avoid communication. But as communicating entails a kind of exertion, so not breathing fully actually inhibits all kinds of productive work. For example, look around you now and locate some fairly heavy object, and pick it up; or unscrew the tightly closed lid of a jar. Then read the next paragraph.

If you are like most people, you took a deep breath, held it, and set your body before lifting the heavy object, or you held your breath at the moment you exerted effort in your hands and arms to open the jar. In either case you immobilized part of your body to provide the illusions of stability and strength. You closed your breath down and actually turned off most of your body in an attempt to focus your energy on those parts with which you were trying to do something.

Now unscrew a tight lid or lift a heavy object *without* holding yourself rigid. Keep breathing through the process of bending and lifting, or grasping and turning: Keep all your motion fluid and notice how your feeling of effort or lack of effort is affected. In a way, knowing something is going to be hard to do inclines us to make ourselves hard as well, by holding our breath. And as we have learned to hold our breath when doing something effortful, so when we hold our breath we automatically tend to exert effort at a task—often far more effort than the task requires.

BREATH AND THE SPIRIT

The physical connection between breath and energy is also a manifestation of the metaphysical qualities of breath, whose influence we experience quite tangibly in the body. In many Oriental systems of thought, breath is called the energy of life, or the life force *(chi* or *prana),* and the Judeo-Christian traditions begin with the premise that God breathed life into Adam.

The word *inspiration* speaks directly to the idea of bringing *in spirit* to the body, and a central concern of breathing well is to fully express the body's ability to integrate and manifest spirit effortlessly. We have said elsewhere in this book that the body is the hologram of the being, and we have observed that here in the physical world we deal with the being through that hologram. In bodywork we expand the horizons of our client's inspiration by freeing the torso from chronic tensions and allowing the movement of breath to regain its naturally deep and fluid rhythms. Inspiration may then move the being, as breath moves the holographic body.

At the beginning of this chapter we asked what inspires you; now we ask a couple of related but distinctly different questions: What does spirituality mean to you? How do you develop spiritually? Do you even want to do so? Does it matter to you?

Over the centuries, many people considering just such questions have concluded that spiritual growth leads to experiences of satisfaction and contentment with life itself, just as learning leads to intellectual pleasures and regular exercise leads to a feeling of bodily well-being. In addition, they have generally found that spiritual growth begins when an increasing amount of energy is permitted to flow through the body—often, though not always, in the form of breath—opening it up as the spirit's channel.

Around the turn of the last century, Emile Durkheim

Bill: I don't know where I got the idea that I was supposed to hold my breath—and subsequently hold my entire body—in order to lift anything, but as a consequence of doing so I used to find all sorts of exercise very stressful and unpleasant. Moreover, I once threw my back out just picking up a shoe, and another time I threw it out doing an exercise that was supposed to make my back stronger and more supple. It was not until I started breathing *through* my physical tasks that I began to find them easy and to enjoy exercising. At the same time, I found I could do far more than I had done before, while exerting far less effort.

Joseph: When I am working with a client and start to exert effort in my breathing for any reason, either by holding my breath or trying to breathe in some way that does not come naturally to me, the rigidity of that breathing is transferred into rigidity in my whole body. As a result I become tired quickly, the quality of my touch becomes irritating to my client, and both the client and I experience a reduction of the energy flow between us. This simple sort of lesson at the physical level can be applied in any aspect of life: It is possible not only to *do* things well with ease, but also just to *be* with ease.

Only when we are reconnected to our bodies can we experience true spirituality.
—attributed to Dora Kalff

Client: My meditation became much deeper [after the first session]. I was able to feel at ease as I sat, and to inhale more deeply.

Client: Until I began the Hellerwork series I regarded myself as a highly spiritual person. I was vegetarian, I had been celibate for over a year. After the first session I started eating meat and moved in with my girlfriend. I still regard myself as spiritual. I just don't have to put on an act about it.

Client: After the first session I was really able to hit the hell out of my golf ball. Partly, I found I was able to breathe through the effort of my swing, and partly I felt more freedom between my rib cage and pelvis, so I could rotate better on the swing.

Fear is excitement without breath.
—Fritz Perls

wrote a book called *The Way of Transformation: Daily Life as a Spiritual Exercise,* whose title embraces both the physical and the metaphysical concerns of this chapter: inspiration embodied in every moment of every thought and act. One of the premises on which Hellerwork is built is that anyone can experience himself as a full manifestation of spirit in the simple acts of daily life without having to retire from the hurley-burley. Because if the only way we could experience our spirituality was by shunning daily life, then most of us would be left with a greater separation, rather than an affirmed unity, between body and spirit.

Through inspiration we can discover the body as an affirmation of the spirit, rather than an impediment to it, a prison for it, a cage in which it is trapped, a machine for the ghost, or anything else that makes the manifestation of spirit more difficult rather than simpler.

Matter seems able to exist in a lifeless state, but breath changes matter from something inert to something vital. As life begins with inspiration, so inspiration is one of the *sine qua non*s of life.

In the conventional Western hospital birth, the new baby is often *made* to take its first breath. The attitude that we should introduce an infant to life by slapping its bottom to "force" it to breathe expresses a cultural assumption most of us have embraced, and which we contest throughout this book: that life is inherently hard, so that you have to hold your breath, grit your teeth, put your shoulder to the wheel, gird your loins, push on through, and bear up under its trials and tribulations.

While children are in school, sooner or later some teacher tells them to study hard, think hard (how does one think hard?), and at some point most kids panic and hold their breath. Fear: excitement without breath. As education instills this attitude in our children they spend a lot of their adult lives (*we* spend a lot of *our* adult lives, because this is what happened to most of us) holding. We hold our bodies tense: We hold on to our limbs and bones, not with our hands but with our musculature; we hold fast to our feelings and thoughts and beliefs and to the very bodily attitudes that in some ways engendered them in the first place.

Tighten your abdomen and inhale. Where do you feel rigid? In other words, where does your inhalation stop? Where will your breath not go? Can you feel the breath pressing out against your chest? Your belly? Does it even reach your abdomen? Can you feel any movement at all in your hips, your shoulders, your neck? Now exhale, relax your abdomen, and take another breath. How far down, up, and throughout your body can you feel movement? Is the movement the air itself that you inhaled? Is it simply the motion of the pressure wave radiating out through your entire being?

Find one place in your body where the first breath did not quite reach, and put the fingers of one hand on that part of your body. Breathe again, mentally aiming the breath toward your fingers. Breathe that way a few times. If you do not actually feel the movement of the breath start to reach your fingers, you probably will feel the gradual softening of the muscles beneath your fingers: a loosening up of your stiffness as you bring the breath down into your own fingertips. If you place your fingers on a part of your body that is experiencing muscular pain, it is very likely the pain will diminish after just a few minutes of such breathing, as you release your hold on the muscles.

In part, what you have just experienced is a result of your own individual learning process, and in part it is something all societies teach all their members from the cradle: how to control energy. A society propagates itself by limiting the expression of individual as well as collective energy to a few permissible areas. Societies therefore

Joseph: When most people think about taking a full breath they think of filling their abdomens. That is because they have tight rib cages that do not move upon inspiration, forcing the diaphragm to press on the abdominal contents. When the rib cage is released, inspiration takes place by the bellows movement of the rib cage. That involves movement in the ribs that can easily be felt and does not press on the abdominal contents.

115

teach people to control their energies by limiting the ways in which, and the degrees to which, they are allowed to express themselves. For instance, it is not all right in any society to fully express open sexuality, nor is it all right to express intense emotions in any but a few circumstances. Rather, we are taught to hold back certain parts of our energy spectrum, just as we are taught not to let our body fluids leak.

Although we are supposed to learn about control as we become socialized, the social view of control is pronouncedly immature, emphasizing restrictions rather than motivations, so that we learn to dam our energies up rather than use them in ways that might benefit both ourselves and others. Instead of learning to expand ourselves to embrace the world, we learn to close ourselves down and close the world out. We learn to hold our breath and live with a minimum of inspiration, when our embodied opportunity is to take the air deeply, free of restrictions on our natural aptitudes for living and being fully, completely inspired.

Client: I used to be frightened of running out of inspiration, as if some well of excitement could dry up on me. But I discovered that inspiration is a physical thing, almost a substance, I could draw upon. I learned I could inspire myself through breathing.

We discussed the problems of breathing with a depressed attitude earlier, when we asked you to hunch yourself over and then talk about something inspiring. A parallel issue of posture and attitude, which creates parallel kinds of breathing difficulties, is the inflation in which a person holds his chest tight and high and thrust forward while holding his shoulders high and his belly in, restricting his breath to his abdomen (this tends to be a male posture of control, popular wherever uniforms are worn).

Try this posture out and see for yourself how your breathing becomes constricted. What happens to your awareness and your ability to respond emotionally? Stand that way and try to feel tender toward someone you love, miss, or long for. The posture is rigid while the emotional tone engendered by these sorts of thoughts is extremely fluid, and the conflicting attitudes are virtually impossible to hold together for long. Either the posture will result in quick, shallow breaths and a rigidification of your thoughts, or it may even banish soft thoughts altogether. Another possibility is that the thoughts themselves will encourage you to breathe more slowly, bringing about a relaxation in your stance.

It is also true that your breathing can control your attitude, rather than the other way around. For instance, if your breathing is hard and shallow while you stand in this position, you will harden your mind and your body at once; by the same token, if you take long, slow, deep breaths, your whole attitude will begin to soften both internally and externally.

Simply in the course of your daily life, you will find you often stop breathing—as, for instance, when you are walking up stairs. Does your breathing hesitate as you start to lift a foot? Or when you shift your weight forward? What about when you bend down to pick up a bag of groceries or a child? When you sit down? In our efforts to conserve energy by holding our breath, we really make our bodies solid, and we lock up our energies and inspiration in them. Particularly when we are in the midst of movement—walking a flight of stairs or picking up a baby —to stop breathing is actually to expend effort rather than conserve it, and to create strain rather than diminish it.

Hellerwork affirms the spiritual value of placing your awareness fully in the embodied moment, in the simple action that is taking place right now, such as the movement entailed in sitting down or brushing your teeth. It affirms the inspiration of every experience, which can be limitlessly wealthy, deep, and broad. And the way into this experience taught by all the yogas, whether by breathing, posture, diet, action, or sex, is directly and explicitly through the body.

Underneath the view that you must leave the material world to experience spirituality lies fear of the body and the belief that inspiration is something special that you must struggle or suffer to achieve. But the simple act of breathing requires no special effort, and similarly no effort is required to become connected with spirit. The body is already an inspired organism, and every moment, from your first breath to your last, is an opportunity to breathe in life's joy and fullness. Inspiration not only includes both breath and spirit, then, but is actually the meeting point at which the two merge; and the unification that takes place in you takes place automatically, unconsciously, effortlessly, and inevitably.

UNDERSTANDING, OR, STANDING ON YOUR OWN TWO FEET

7

THE FEET AND LEGS

Notice what your feet are doing. Notice the position they are in, notice what they feel like, notice what you did with them as you read the first words in this chapter: Did they become tight or loose, move or stay still? One thing you probably found is that your feet were not on the ground. You were either leaning on the sides of your feet or you had one leg crossed over the other and one foot dangling in mid-air, or your feet may have been up on a desk or couch, or you may have had them standing on their toes, or perhaps you were sitting on one leg. One thing, however, is almost certain: You did not have both feet planted firmly on the floor, and it is virtually certain that you almost never have.

To take this experiment a step further, stand up and notice whether your weight is more heavily placed on one foot than on the other. Many people who may not stand back on their heels or up on their toes ordinarily stand instead with their weight primarily on one leg, the opposing knee slightly bent, and its corresponding hip raised. Like most of our habitual postures, such a supposedly casual position reflects the tension of some kind of misalignment—an imbalance in the hips, for instance. In other words, our postures reflect our failure to understand our bodies. Just what is it that stands under what?

KEEPING YOUR FEET ON THE GROUND

Most of the terms we use to signify intelligence concern the hands: grasp, handle, hold. The compound word *under-stand* is the only one that concerns the feet and it is the one that suggests that knowledge needs a foundation in order to be useful. If the temperature is 60 degrees Fahrenheit, is it hot or cold? Well, hot or cold for what? For August in the tropics? For January in Alaska? For boiling an egg? For making ice? The number by itself is meaningless unless we understand the concept of tem-

Client: My hands and feet used to fall asleep quite frequently, but since the second session they no longer seem to do so. Since I have also been experiencing a tingling in my feet, I presume the session improved my circulation as well as increasing my awareness of my connection with the Earth.

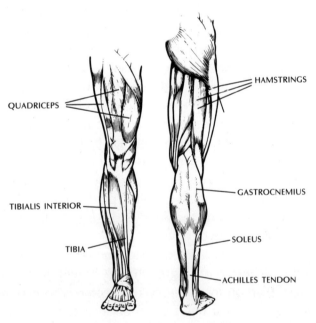

Figure 7-1. The superficial muscles of the leg: front (l) and back (r).

perature, understand what the Fahrenheit scale implies, and understand relative thermal values. Understanding provides the foundation for turning mere information into knowledge, and ultimately for turning knowledge into wisdom. And the physical counterpart of understanding is having your feet planted firmly on the ground.

To be firmly grounded means you are in good contact with the Earth—that your weight is both evenly and easily distributed over your two feet, reflecting a structure in balance from top to bottom and from side to side. If you look at the bottoms of your feet, however, you will find callouses here, corns and bunions there. These growths appear in places where the connective tissues have hardened in order to protect themselves from the exertion of more weight or pressure than they were designed to bear. Your shoes do not generate new tissue in the same way your body does, and if you look at their

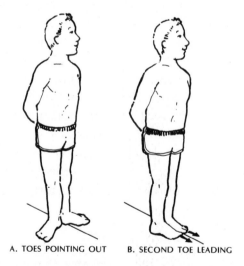

A. TOES POINTING OUT   B. SECOND TOE LEADING

Figure 7-2. Many people stand and walk with their weight traveling forward at an angle through their feet, while the weight of their bodies actually moves forward. (A) The imbalanced movement creates stress throughout the physical structure. Ideally (B), your weight travels forward in a straight line from the middle of your heel through the midline of your foot and on into your second toe. The flowing movement that results reflects the balanced design of your body's structure.

soles you will find that whereas some areas are conspicuously worn, others are nearly untouched by the ground you walk on.

Except for the arch, which normally does not touch the ground, the bottom of your shoe should—ideally—be worn fairly evenly, reflecting a balanced pressure that, in turn, reflects a general condition of balance throughout the body. If parts of your shoe bottom do not touch the ground it is because they cannot get there. When the physical structure above is out of balance, its imbalance is *always,* with no exceptions, reflected in the way its weight is distributed in the foot.

Take a walk across the room right now, and notice how the weight of your body travels through your foot as you move. Everybody's foot touches the ground heel first. Ideally, your weight then travels forward in a straight path from the middle of your heel through the midline of your foot and on into your second toe. This flowing movement reflects the balanced design of your body's structure. But the ideal is not common in the modern world. For instance, as you walked you may have found your weight moving on the inside edges of your feet; or, more likely, you found your weight traveling around the outer edge of your foot in a semicircular fashion, sweeping wide from your heel to end up in your big toe as you were ready to take your next step. These common sorts of rigid movements reflect the misaligned functioning—the imbalance—of your body's structure.

Client: Learning to walk and learning to stand have made an enormous difference in my work [as a bartender]. Because I am better balanced all around, I no longer become fatigued on the job.

THE STRUCTURE OF THE FOOT

The foot is the foundation through which the body transfers its weight to the ground. In this regard, its first function is to provide a stable base where the body's weight shifts from an essentially vertical pole to a horizontal platform. The foot is able to effect this transfer because

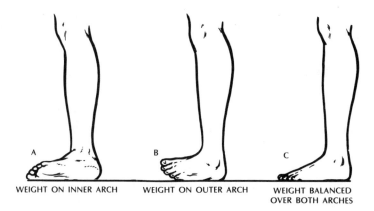

A — WEIGHT ON INNER ARCH   B — WEIGHT ON OUTER ARCH   C — WEIGHT BALANCED OVER BOTH ARCHES

Figure 7-3. People frequently stand and walk with their weight on the inner or outer arches of their feet, resulting in rigid postures and rigid walking movements. When the body is in balance, its weight is balanced over both arches.

of its construction, which is basically triangular. The triangle is the most stable simple structural unit in nature, and the pyramid, which is based on the triangle, is the simplest three-dimensional form that allows for the transfer of a vertical force onto a horizontal base. A four-sided pyramid (three face-sides and a base), known as a tetrahedron, is the simplest three-dimensional pyramid—hence, the simplest three-dimensional structural unit known. And this is what the foot is: a tetrahedron whose base is a triangle formed by the back of the heel, the small toe, and the large toe. The third dimension of the tetrahedron of the foot is created by the top of the ankle bone, called the talus.

The foot's second function is to allow for walking, which is accomplished through its three arches. The largest and best-known of the foot's arches is the *medial* arch, which forms the hollow at the "palm" of the foot. The smaller, *lateral* arch lies parallel to the medial arch on the outside of the foot, and the *transverse* arch reaches across the foot immediately behind the toes. The

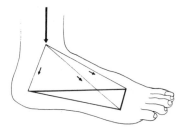

Figure 7-4. The foot as a tetrahedron.

123

Joseph: When I began my journey into bodywork I was extremely flat-footed—so much so that when I walked in wet sand I not only made an imprint that had no indentation at all on its inner side, but actually made a little bulge where my ankle collapsed inward. And I was very, very unaware of any kind of connection with the ground. After some bodywork, I developed a real arch: Nothing to write home about, but now there's a small indentation in my footprint, and my walk is much more springy, flexible, and elastic. My arches do their work as suspension mechanisms instead of letting my feet plod along, flop, flop, flop.

arches absorb shock, allowing the entire organism to move along the ground with a maximum of ease and a minimum of discomfort. At the same time, they contribute to the foot's enormous strength and flexibility. As we know from building architectural structures, the arch—itself based on the triangle—is one of the strongest structural units ever devised; and, like arches in bridges, doorways, and other bearing structures, the arches of the foot are designed to support heavy loads by spreading their weight out over a span larger than the column that feeds the arch.

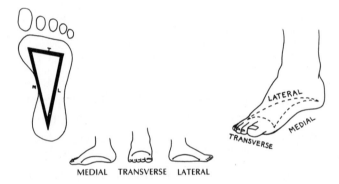

MEDIAL   TRANSVERSE   LATERAL

Figure 7-5. The arches of the foot.

It is not quite enough to say that the arches contribute to the foot's flexibility, although they do; but they are also designed to maximize the foot's *stability* through that flexibility. If you examine the bony structures of the hands and feet, you will find them remarkably similar. Both are organized to allow for the same sorts of movement, and intrinsically our feet have almost as much movement capability as our hands. Babies curling their feet in their cribs demonstrate the inherent flexibility of these structures, and so do some arm amputees, who learn to do with their feet virtually everything the rest of us do with our hands, including write, paint, drive, and eat.

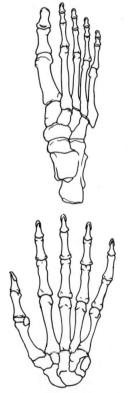

Figure 7-6. Bones of the hand and foot showing similarity of structure.

Most of us lost the innate flexibility of our feet long ago. When we started to stand on our own two feet, our structures began to rigidify in response to the imbalanced weight loads we imposed, and this rigidity has contributed to the imbalance ever since. Moreover, the imbalance contributed to the rigidity in a self-perpetuating circle of deteriorating function.

The weight of the body itself was never the problem, but rather it was the imbalance that naturally inclined us to tighten up as we tried to right ourselves. We can see babies do that with their feet as they learn to stand and walk. If you have ever walked a tightrope or a rail you probably became aware that your feet were actually tensing as they tried to grip the narrow surface, even if you were wearing shoes at the time. But that tightening process, which is transitory at first, became permanent as our bodies adapted to the functional realities of our physical lives.

If you ever have the opportunity to visit a tropical island, you will see that the feet of those natives who still go barefoot are much more flexible than ours. Even though these people go through the same processes we do of learning to stand and walk when they are small, their feet do not become permanently crippled as a result. A native Tahitian climbs a coconut tree by wrapping his hands *and his feet* around the tree's trunk, and simply walking up the tree. He can also change the height of his medial arches when walking over rocks and uneven terrain, a movement the foot is designed to perform but which is entirely foreign to most of us who live in industrialized countries.

In the developed world, we mostly walk on surfaces that are uniformly hard and uniformly flat. Of course, there is some difference between walking on concrete and walking on a shag rug, and our cities and towns have hills and driveways and even little bumps in the road. But

Bill: I'm particularly interested in your story, since my own experience is exactly opposite. I have very high arches, arches ballet dancers hate me for. Years ago a friend noticed that I tended to spring up on my toes when I walked, and I recognized the connection between my walk, my arches, and what was then my fervent desire not to exist on this planet, not to be in this world. As I went through Rolfing and Hellerwork my arches did not get any flatter, but they did get more pliable, so that when I walk more of my arch comes down and more of my foot touches the ground. Although I am not quite willing to say that bodywork was the sole cause of this change, I no longer want to bounce off into the heavens: I have somehow become quite satisfied with being on this Earth.

Joseph: I once worked on a seventy-five-year-old man who had had a club foot from birth. His lower leg, ankle, and foot were severely atrophied, almost literally skin and bones. In the course of the sessions those tissues literally revived, and he grew muscles in his calves and acquired movement in his ankles that he had never had before.

these sorts of variations are insignificant compared with the yielding depths of sandy shores, leafy forest floors, and springy marshes and meadows, or with the variable surfaces where stones and shells and pinecones and rocks, anthills, gopher holes, and fallen tree limbs meet the feet at every turning.

In primitive societies, people have to adapt themselves constantly to the changing surfaces of their world. In doing so they use the bones as well as the muscles of their feet to keep their balance. As a result they constantly exercise their feet, which remain flexible. On as flat a surface as a hardwood floor or a concrete sidewalk, however, no such demands are made of the feet: The artificial surface provides adequate support for balance, and the complex structures of the feet get set in their easy ways. The foot turns into a paddle, and its tissues rigidify into a pad.

Where our floors fail to reduce the adaptability of our feet, our shoes pick up the slack in two ways. First, they almost all have heels that throw our bodies forward, concentrating our weight toward the front of our feet rather than distributing it evenly throughout the horizontal surface. By forcing us out of balance in this way, our shoes effectively demand that we lean backward to compensate for our imbalance, which accounts for the fact that most of us wear out the heels of our shoes at a relatively rapid rate. Second, the shapes of our shoes resemble the shapes of our feet very little. They are usually designed to squeeze the foot, particularly at the toe, into a narrow, highly unnatural form, thereby eliminating almost all of whatever movement potential remains to these once-dynamic appendages.

Whether a cause, an effect, or merely a coincidence of humanity's strange floor and shoe customs, most courtly and urban cultures in the world, from Europe to China, have held small feet in high esteem. It is virtually a worldwide stereotype among advanced nations that people with small feet and high arches are aristocratic, do not have to work with their bodies, and ride from place to place, whereas people with large feet and low or flat arches are peasants who do physical labor and must walk when they have somewhere to go. As a result, the damage we do to our feet simply in the course of living in society is compounded by our cultural assumption that what we are doing is desirable. Because it is so much a part of our daily lives, the system that de-feets us is hard to beat, or even to perceive. Meanwhile, of course, it makes the fact that we remain mobile at all a remarkable testament to human fortitude.

While our feet are putting up with all these direct assaults on their integrity they must also contend with imbalance in the higher reaches of the human structure, because they are the court of last resort in keeping our swaying forms more or less upright as we lurch and stagger through the world. If you consider the human edifice as a tall tower balanced on a small base, you can see that as soon as the tower leans in any direction its weight can no longer be distributed evenly over that whole base, but must become concentrated in an increasingly small area. In the preceding chapter we talked about balancing the chest over the pelvis. The next phase in balancing the body is to bring that balanced weight of the torso down onto the ground.

THE LEG AND ITS JOINTS:
THE ANKLE AND THE KNEE

Among all the joints of the body, the ankle is subject to unique pressures. Ponder the case of a 180-pound man standing still. Less the incidental pounds his feet weigh, each of his ankles is supporting 90 pounds on a cross-section of tissue about three square inches in size. At rest, doing nothing, his ankles withstand a pressure of 30 pounds per square inch, or 4,320 pounds per square foot.

When he starts to move, the instantaneous pressure on his ankles at the moment of impact when each foot strikes the ground is several times as great. And when he runs or jumps down from a high place, each of his ankles may support a pressure that has been estimated (by *National Geographic,* in its "Man the Magnificent Machine") as high as *10,000* pounds per square inch.

Most people encounter ankle problems at some time in their lives. Twists, sprains, and strains are common, and result as much from rigidity that prevents the joint from accommodating pressure as from the effects of pressure itself. For some people, compression over the years results in a chronic thickening of the tissues. This compression is a result of imbalance higher up in the body.

Above the ankle, the knee performs the most delicate of all the body's mechanical balancing acts, keeping

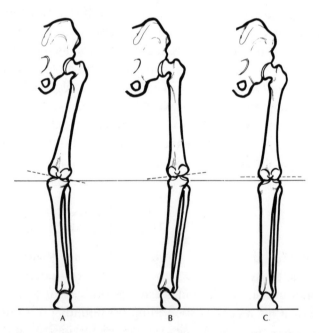

Figure 7-7. The knee joint in gravity. (A) knock knees; (B) bowed legs; (C) aligned legs.

one long, heavy stick in position above another long, somewhat narrower stick. The knee joint can be in equilibrium only at one precise place, which is in direct alignment with gravity. Any deviation from that alignment shoves the knee out of balance. And when the knee falls out of balance, carrying the weight of most of the body with it, we tighten muscles from the scalp to the toes in an effort to remain standing upright. One of the most frequent and observable reactions to imbalance at the knee is hyperextension of the joint: "locking" the knee and holding it rigidly in place in an attempt to achieve stability.

If you have a willing companion handy, stand facing him or her at arm's length, and lock your knees. Now ask your partner to push you gently from in front. You will discover that very little pressure is enough to make you topple backward. If you are alone, you can push yourself off from a wall with the same result. With your knees locked you become unstable, a pushover, weak-kneed, unable to hold your ground. Such is the price of rigidity. If you try the same experiment with your knees loose, you will find the push is buffered and absorbed in the knee joint, and that you can absorb a great deal more force without losing your balance.

Whenever we feel unstable we tense up (or compress) somewhere in our bodies. By doing this we achieve exactly the opposite of what we intended: Instead of making ourselves *more* stable we make ourselves *less* stable. The feeling of instability that makes us tense up need not be physical. Although walking a shaky plank over a high chasm will bring the lesson home immediately and impressively, it can be derived equally well from feelings of psychological or mental instability, as Reich, Lowen, and others have pointed out. Gripping psychologically or mentally can lead to emotional and mental rigidities in the same way that gripping physically leads to physical rigidities. Moreover, physical rigidities lead to psychological rigidities, and psychological rigidities lead to physical rigidities. Because the human being is an integrated system, gripping in *any* realm will affect stability in *every* realm. This is easiest to see, of course, and easiest to address, in the body.

When a person takes a truly balanced stance, her legs go straight down under her torso, and her feet are as wide apart as her hip joints. From the front, this ideal alignment shows the hip joint positioned over the knee joint, the knee joint over the ankle joint, and the ankle joint over the foot in a smooth vertical line. But as she experiences more and more instability in her physical, emotional, or mental life, she will tend to spread her feet farther apart in an A-frame configuration, in an attempt to widen her base of support. What this means, of course, is that someone standing with her feet wide apart feels unstable.

You have probably recognized that the classic A-

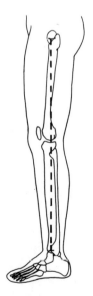

Figure 7-8. Ideal leg alignment.

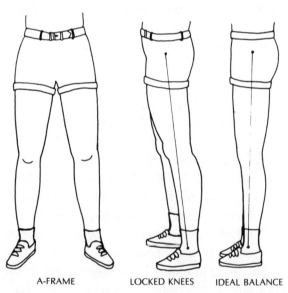

A-FRAME   LOCKED KNEES   IDEAL BALANCE

Figure 7-9. A-frame instability.

frame tough-guy pose not only defeats its own purpose —to show that one can hold one's ground against attack —but even proclaims one's vulnerability. There is some justification for taking the stance as a way of *gaining* stability, in that it forms a triangle under the body, which is inherently more stable than the rectangle effected by a simple up-and-down posture. But this is an issue of effect only. Since the legs are hinged, rather than unitary, the farther apart you spread them, the more you will find you have to lock your knees to maintain your posture. And as we have seen, locked knees defeat their own purpose and produce imbalance throughout the human structure.

The knees are not designed to be unstable, of course: They are unstable as a consequence of their design value, which is flexibility. On top of these joints rests the whole weight of the trunk, which is distributed onto the two legs through the pelvis. The knees' flexibility allows them to buffer imbalances from higher up, keeping the body erect when by all rights it should be lying in a heap; but knees may be forced do so at the expense of their own integrity, as well as that of the ankles and feet, if they allow the upper body to adapt to its imbalances rather than making integral corrections.

If you have two bathroom scales that are about equally accurate, stand with one foot on either scale while looking straight ahead. When you think you are well balanced, ask someone to read the weights on the two scales for you. We suggest using a second person because you will tend to lean in the direction of the scale you're reading, whichever that may be, and will miss the point of this little experiment. If you are alone, take care to simply lower your head straight down when you read the numbers. Obviously, the total weight is not our concern here. The question is, how much difference is there between the weights your two legs are supporting?

WALKING

As we have noted, any rigidity diminishes the entire body's ability to move. Most people do not experience all the restrictions their habits engender, because they move within a fairly restricted range of space by the time they have grown up. For the average person, for instance, the act of simply walking does not begin to put the structures of the foot and leg through their paces. In average walking—what most of us do most of the time—the ankle joint tenses slightly and then stresses slightly, moving through a modest range of perhaps 90 degrees. But in normal walking—what most of us are designed to be capable of—the trailing foot will bend nearly 180 degrees at the moment the toes of that foot leave the ground.

If you watch a horse walk, you will see that its ankle is loose and holds no tension; when you watch the foot-loose natives of some South Seas atoll walk, you see the same thing: The foot drops as the ankle extends, and it straightens as the ankle flexes, in a process quite distinct from ours. We wear shoes, which restrict the ankle's mobility; we wear sandals or backless thongs, which demand that we tense our toes and flex our feet to keep the shoe substitutes horizontal when they touch the ground; we wear boots and hightop basketball shoes, which are explicitly designed to prevent ankle movement and to protect our ankles from the perils of, say, falling from stirrups and saddle or pivoting suddenly on a basketball court. But none of our sophisticated footgear does much to support or accommodate what our feet are designed to do, which is simply to enable us to move from place to place.

What is true for the ankle is no less true for the knee. Whereas the knee is capable of practically 180 degrees of flection, most people—particularly women in high heels and men in riding boots—walk as if on stilts and

132

rarely extend their knees beyond about 50 degrees. This rigid, stilted form of walking makes us move as if we are falling forward.

Stand still, as relaxed and balanced as you can be, and lean your weight forward so that your head moves in front of your feet. You will not get very far before the momentum of your weight starts to make you move your feet; otherwise you'll fall flat on your face. This is the way most of us walk, as if we are trying to get ahead in life. We move by falling, and our legs are always trying to catch up.

Now stand still again, relaxed as before. Rather than leaning ahead, move one knee forward and transfer your weight to that foot; as you put the foot down, move your back knee forward and transfer your weight to *that* foot. In this kind of locomotion you carry your torso with your legs. Not only do your joints have an opportunity to exercise themselves, but your entire motion becomes fluid and graceful and relaxed—balanced, in a word. Even when you lift one knee you remain balanced on the foot that is still on the ground. You can even walk this way in slow motion, as mimes do when they want to imitate a walk, and you can stop in midstep without falling over, because you are entirely with yourself: There is nothing to catch up to.

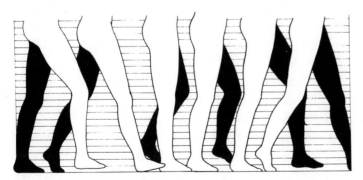

Figure 7-10. Proper movements of the leg in simple walking.

STANDING UP FOR YOURSELF

The way we habitually move reflects our willingness to stand on our own two feet, to have our feet on the ground, to take a stand, to have standing in our families, professions, and communities, to have standards, to be upstanding, to stand for something. Our language reflects our relationships with our bodies in the same way that our bodies reflect our relationships with everyday reality, so that having your feet on the ground implies something quite different from walking on air or having your head in the clouds. Our use of language literally communicates to us about our willingness to be in touch with reality. And the way in which we deal with everyday reality reflects our ability to take care of ourselves, or in other words, to be independent.

To be independent is to stand on your own two feet. It is an ability that distinguishes the utterly helpless infant from the child who can walk to the refrigerator, the bathroom, the toy chest, the bookshelf, the television set.

Independence does not mean being unable to depend on others, however. In modern society we are all dependent on each other, our lives intertwined with those of millions of other people who provide us with electricity, oil, food, clothing, roads, cars, markets, and so forth. Independence means the ability to take care of ourselves, to stand up for ourselves within the framework our culture provides. And at this level, independence demands the ability to move.

"Standing on your own two feet," "keeping your feet on the ground," "taking a stand," and other colloquial expressions all address the subject of grounding. Grounding means allowing energy to flow between us and the ground beneath us. In one sense, this flow of energy can make us well grounded in a subject we want to understand; in another, it is how we become rooted and come to feel that we belong somewhere. As our clichés suggest, people who are grounded tend to walk firmly, feet first, with ease and balance, while those who are up in the clouds seem to lead with their heads. In some ways we live in a head-oriented culture that values addressing abstract concepts in a rational fashion. Yet we also value thinking on our feet.

To think on one's feet implies that one is mentally agile and capable of processing information rapidly while under pressure. This is an essential ability not only for some professions—football quarterback, for example, or emergency room physician—but it may also be an essential ability for day-to-day living. Most of us think on our rear ends, which means that we separate thinking from acting. We say, "Let's think about this," and sit around a table analyzing whatever "this" may be until we feel prepared to go into action and *do* something about it. Often we then act without giving the matter further thought, even though circumstances may change that would argue for a newly thought-out course of action.

To conclude this chapter, we would like you to experience the ease of balanced walking. First, walk about the room in the most usual, everyday fashion you can. Notice the amount of effort you exert, and the amount of shock you experience in your whole structure as you move. Notice the impact on your body when your heels strike the floor, notice the way your torso sways and the way your hips move or do not move in order to keep it upright. Notice any tension in or around your knees; notice any stress in or around your ankles. Notice what you do with your shoulders, neck, and head to help you maintain your equilibrium. Notice any tightness, particularly in your jaw or abdomen.

When you think you have some sense of what your own walking is like, stop and reposition yourself. Stand in as relaxed a manner as you can, with your feet side by

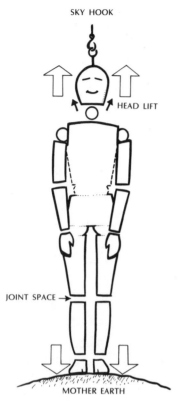

Figure 7-11. Using the sky hook.

side, and when you feel fairly stable, slowly begin to rock forward and back from your ankles. Zero in on the position in which your weight is evenly distributed between the ball and the heel of your foot: where it feels as though your weight comes down from your body through the center of your ankle. When you have that position well in hand—or in foot—unlock your knees.

Imagine that the top of your head is suspended from what Ida Rolf used to call a *sky hook* (see illustration), and begin to walk as if that hook were holding you up, so that you can let your shoulders, arms, spine, back, hips, and legs just hang along with you. Now move one knee forward and let it down; then move the other knee forward and let *it* down. As you walk about the room, notice how much more evenly your weight is distributed over your feet than it was before and how much more softly your feet strike the floor. As you walk, let the arches of your feet relax and feel springy. Let your ankles stay loose, let your knees be soft, and relax your hip joints. Now observe that when you take care to have your body balanced and relaxed, walking can become a truly effortless activity.

REACHING OUT

8

THE ARMS AND SIDES

We discussed the torso in Chapter 6, "Inspiration," and the legs and feet in Chapter 7, "Understanding." This chapter about the arms and sides completes our exploration of the body's superficial musculature. "Reaching Out" also completes one of this book's developmental sequences: As breath precedes self-awareness, so a person must be capable of standing on his own before he can truly reach out to others, or else he would topple from imbalance and be capable only of leaning on someone else. "Inspiration" concerns your relationship with spirit, then, "Understanding" is about your relationship with yourself, and "Reaching Out" entails your relationships with other people.

ARMS AND THE HUMAN

Have you ever noticed how differently various people hold their arms? Yet we all have the same physiology. The arms are connected to the rest of the body through the

137

shoulder girdle, which consists of the clavicles, shoulder blades, and scapulae. The shoulder girdle functions on the principle of a yoke. This yoke, suspended from the muscles of the neck, rests atop the sternum above the rib cage. From it the arms depend, balanced somewhat as a pair of hanging buckets are balanced at the ends of a bamboo stick laid across the shoulders of the water carrier in old Chinese pictures.

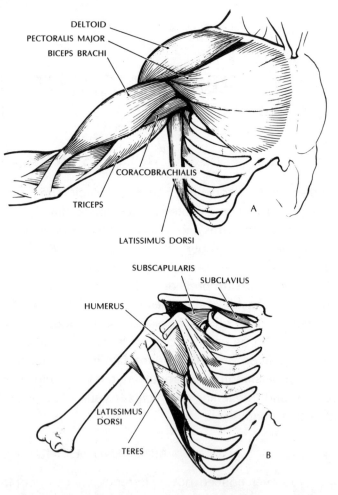

Figure 8-1. Muscles of the shoulder girdle, including arms and chest. Superficial musculature (A) and deep musculature (B).

The way the shoulder girdle is organized, there should be no need to *do* anything to enable the shoulders and arms to hang as they are designed to hang, without rigidities, twists, or attitudes. The elbows should angle laterally away from the center of the body while the palms of the hands face to the back, as we can see they do on our primate cousins in the zoo.

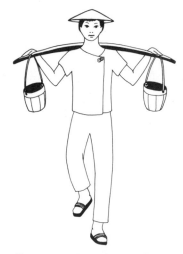

Figure 8-2. Chinese water carrier.

But in fact most people chronically hold their arms and hands in various unnatural ways, rarely allowing them to simply dangle like buckets off the ends of their yoked and balanced shoulders. Our arms are involved in almost everything we do, and, as we have mentioned before, people tend to put a lot of effort into doing things. It should come as no surprise, then, that our arms embody much of the tension that results from effort, or that we frequently express that effort and tension in the ways we use our arms and shoulders, or that we suffer from arthritis, tendonitis, bursitis, dislocations, sprains, and general aches and pains from our fingertips to our shoulders and beyond.

Some of the things we do with our arms are entirely fitting, of course. For example, we raise our shoulders in response to fear, which is an appropriate, natural reaction of the organism when it senses danger. If you are walking down a dark alley and notice that your shoulders are high you might wonder whether there is danger actually present (in which case you might want to leave the alley in a hurry) or whether you are responding out of habit to your belief that dark alleys are dangerous (in which case you might want to relax and enjoy your walk). But if you find your shoulders wrapped around your ears in circumstances that are clearly safe, such as while you're shopping or going to the neighborhood movie theatre to see a comedy with your family, you might wonder whether and/or why you are constantly expecting life to rain blows upon your back. You will not have to wonder why

Client: For as long as I can remember my left arm has been two inches shorter than my right. I have always had my clothing altered accordingly, to make the sleeves look even. After our third session my arms were the same length. Was I amazed? I kept checking in the mirror every day, but eventually I had to admit my clothes no longer fit. I guess that's one of the dangers of bodywork.

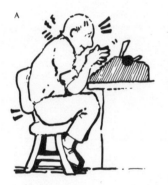

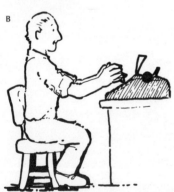

Figure 8-3. Using the shoulders to create tension throughout the body (A), and relaxing the shoulders with the body (B).

your shoulders get tired easily or why your neck feels stiff: You will already have found the answer.

As our individual psycho-physiologies are influenced by the culture in which we live, many people imagine that physical strength is a function of the size of a person's shoulders and arms. This is exactly the kind of misconception that leads to a limited, unbalanced experience of the human body. To some degree, physical strength *is* predicated on the development of the extrinsic musculature; but if someone with huge arms carries them on skinny, stiltlike legs, his big upper body rests on a very unstable base of support. This person may have a great deal of *potential* strength, but be functionally weak because he is too imbalanced to stand his ground, deliver a blow, or to lift or push or pull effectively. Because of the ways in which most of us have adapted ourselves to both personal and social demands for superficial powers, we often exert unnecessary effort to accomplish our ordinary tasks; and the concomitant rigidities of the shoulders and arms are almost universal conditions felt by people who seek relief through bodywork.

SIDE BY SIDE

As the arms hang down from the yoke of the shoulder girdle, they are supported not only by the shoulder joints and the soft tissue of the armpits, but also by that much-ignored part of the body, the sides. Like the seams that join the front of a sweater to its back, the sides are subject to many of the tensions that restrict breathing and other essential body movements. These restrictions come about in part because tension on the sides tightens the rib cage and pulls it down into the pelvis. As a result, the sides actually become shorter, and people bulge beneath the rib cage at their hips with the accumulations of flesh we euphemistically call "love handles." Once the pressure on the sides has been released, however, some portion of these love handles may vanish as the person regains mobility in her trunk, in her ability to reach sideways, and especially in her lateral breathing. The rib cage and the sternum, freed of tension, can then expand out from the body's core as they are designed to do.

Colloquial phrases such as "which side are you on?" and "we're standing side by side" indicate the way we understand the relationship of the sides to the arms. Words pertaining to the sides generally have to do with

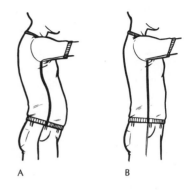

Figure 8-5. Like the seams that join the front of a sweater to its back, the sides are subject to many of the tensions that restrict breathing and other essential body movements. Misaligned sides (A) result in bulges and imbalances in the body; after the sides are aligned they contribute to the body's overall integrity (B).

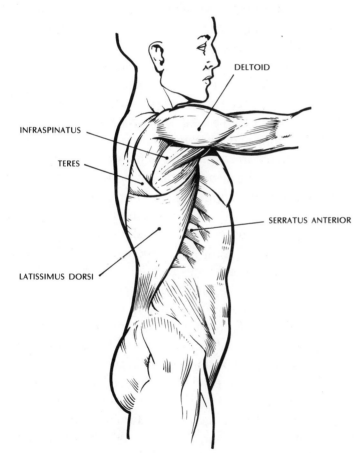

Figure 8-4. Principal muscles of the side.

141

support, and support for the arms is exactly what the sides provide.

After the third session of Hellerwork some people report that they are engaged in a battle with their own shoulders. They consciously let their arms relax, and then three minutes later notice their shoulders have crept back to where they were before the session. But these people are not losing anything at all, except an old, debilitating habit: They have just become aware of the process of physical change. As they become conscious of the effort and tension they hold in their upper limbs, people become increasingly able to liberate the accumulated energy, and they accomplish more while exerting less effort. Eventually the new habit of flexibility sets in.

The well-balanced person exerts as much effort in doing things as necessary, but no more. She has the ability to reach out with ease to shake hands, hug, share love and affection, and be a touching person who touches simply as a natural expression of her desire to make contact with life. She also has the ability to draw back from that which is not appealing, and to push back—to keep things at arm's length—when she feels imposed upon. As we will see in subsequent chapters, restraining aggression in the arms is an extrinsic component of holding back.

As a person becomes aware of the fluctuating tensions in his arms, he may find he needs to pay attention only to what his arms are doing to get a reading on the state of his tension: Tight shoulders and arms imply a tight attitude toward whatever is going on; hanging loose suggests a greater relaxation. In this way the body may be understood as nature's premier biofeedback device. It is a vast storehouse of knowledge that is ours for the asking. It is said that Roman generals, returning from successful campaigns, were given the equivalent of our tickertape parades. As they rode down the streets in their victory chariots, acknowledging the accolades of the crowds,

Joseph: Even after I had learned to relax most of the rest of my body, I still held effort in my arms. As a bodyworker I would try to transfer my weight through my arms into my hands and then into my client's body, but I found I could only lean on my arms to do that if they were stiff as pikes. Then I became more sophisticated and learned to loosen my arms, but my wrists stayed taut; after another while my wrists surrendered but my hands held out since, as I thought, *something* had to be hard to make contact with my client's flesh. But in the past few years I have even been able to let go of my fingers. I discovered that I do not need any rigidity to work with the body's tissues. In fact, the more rigid I am when I touch my client, the more rigid my client becomes in response. My client's rigidity is the *embodiment* of his or her resistance to my own tension. Of course, the tighter my client's muscles, the harder our work becomes. At the same time, when I am loose my client can be loose as well, and we can easily accomplish the work we have come together to perform.

their slaves would stand behind them whispering in their ears, "You are mortal, you are mortal, you are mortal." The body provides similar reminders of who and what and where we are, whatever our beliefs may be.

Take a moment now to consider how your own arms hang when you are standing and at rest. You might even like to pretend you are a gorilla. As you thump around scratching at yourself, you will automatically start to use your arms in a caricature of the way nature designed them to be used; and so, by aping the ape you can start to compare this more or less natural arm posture with the one you habitually employ. What differences do you discern?

Most people carry their arms in a way that reflects who or what they believe they are supposed to be— something other primates do not seem much concerned about. Many of us were raised with injunctions to stand up straight and hold our shoulders back, or otherwise present through our arms the attitudes and images we were taught to express. As a result of our collective acculturation, most of our ideas of what it means to be manly or womanly can be read very easily in the ways we hold and use our arms. And what underlies all these attitudes is the central issue of aggression.

UP IN ARMS

Aggression can be either positive or negative. We are familiar with its negative forms: anger, hostility, violence. It is no accident that nations refer to their weapons as "arms," and it seems fairly certain that bodily arms were what humans first used as weapons. We are also familiar with positive aggression in the form of assertion, although we may not be accustomed to thinking in terms of aggression when we make contact with others, greet, hug, embrace, or simply reach out for what we want.

Relieved of its cultural implications, aggression might

Bill: About fifteen years ago, during a period of enormous personal stress, I was walking around a university campus in New York City and abruptly found that I was able to not hold my shoulders up in either a defensive or an aggressive posture. And as they fell—as I let go of them, and of the tension that had been keeping them in place—I realized that I had been walking around with my shoulders up this way for as long as I could remember. For hours? Weeks? Years, most likely. My relief was so great I wept for twenty minutes.

best be understood as a mutual exchange of complementary, rather than opposing, energies. Seen this way it may not only be difficult to determine which of two people is giving and which receiving, but it is apparent that one form of aggression cannot fully exist without the other.

Manifestations of negative aggression are generally discouraged in our society, with the result that many people who hold tension in their arms also pull their arms back rather than letting them just hang free. In this position the elbows are held behind the body's midline, and the movement of the arms in walking takes place mostly below the elbows. Carried to an extreme and combined with an inflated, forward-thrusting chest, this familiar male attitude is immediately recognizable as the stereotypical pose of the pugnacious street bully or assertive military drill instructor. It is a presentation of self that so radiates an aggressive potential for explosive violence that it warns others instantly to be wary, and keeps them from reaching out.

Related influences provoke a complementary set of attitudes traditionally displayed by women in our society, although they are seen less these days than in the past. In this order of things, good little girls who are to become nice little ladies are taught not to push, hit, climb, throw, carry, lift, or otherwise make powerful use of their arms. By restraining their native aggression they often develop arms that are, in effect, partly atrophied. They grow up with arms that are weak and either flabby or wilted looking. Along with their withheld aggression, such women may, in addition, develop a body posture in which their arms are pulled around with the elbows held close to the sides while the hands face forward—the classic posture of submission.

Try out both these standard, 20th-century, Western poses—the bully and the submissive—for yourself. As you adopt each position, consider the feelings they bring up for you: not just the feelings immediately associated with each stance, but also the feelings the first feelings evoke. For many people, the bully posture initially manifests as anger, rage, and the urge to strike, but under these feelings you may find a great cowering fear and a desire to run or to be held and comforted. The submissive posture, on the other hand, frequently engenders a desire to yield, to fall back, to give up; but often, beneath these so-called feminine feelings, an enormous rage is seething against the demands of inhibition. During Hellerwork, the client has a chance to explore the feelings on the surface of the pose, to learn their value, and to find out something of the emotional price he or she pays by repressing the feelings that lie underneath them. Clients also start to learn the value inherent in the feelings they have held down, and the power of the energy that is released when they start to include them in their emotional repertoire.

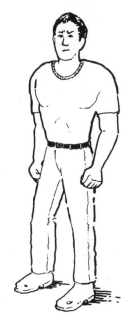

Figure 8-6. The street bully: dominant posture.

You might try to perform a few simple actions from your own day-to-day life while holding these picturesque positions. Try, for example, to run or throw a ball or even to reach out to lift some little object while holding your arms in what used to be a common female attitude, and feel how greatly the posture impedes any powerful force of your arms. Then, in the bully pose, try to cradle some object tenderly, or with your fingertips pick up a fragile flower, and feel how greatly that stance restricts your ability to be receptive to what you desire.

If you have a chance to experiment with another person, you can also try reaching out to him or her in different ways—softly, angrily, and so on—while holding your arms in each of these two postures, in order to understand some of the ways in which we succeed and fail in being both positively and negatively aggressive with each other.

Aggression is one of the areas in life where we experience enormous stress, not only because our arms are

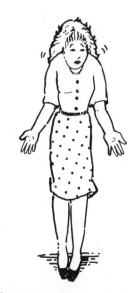

Figure 8-7. Submissive posture.

Client: Two days after my session on the arms I was suddenly able to express anger to my husband. I don't mean I reached out and hit him, but I let my body posture demonstrate my feelings. I felt my shoulders go up and my elbows tuck in and I clenched my fists. I sort of backed away from him and bent down over my belly as if protecting my soft parts from blows, and then I told him how I felt. I had always been afraid that if I expressed my anger either I would go out of control and become a screaming fury, or else that he would hate me for it. But instead, things got a lot more real between us. I was able to let go of my anger after I spoke out, and he understood immediately. Later we sat down and had a good talk about all the things that had gone wrong in the past year that we had not been able to discuss till then, and cleared up mountains of garbage from our relationship. With all the energy we freed up we made love until three in the morning.

involved in practically all our activities or because we express a great deal of effort through them, but also because we are often afraid of our aggressive impulses: afraid that if we reach out we may cause pain, or be rebuffed, or end up stuck with what we grasp. One response to such a fear is to refrain from action; another is to overstate the fear.

Next time you are driving or writing or using a small tool of any sort, notice how you tend to tighten your whole arm or both your arms, and how you set your shoulders to deal with whatever little task has come to hand, even when the actual labor involved may require no more exertion than you could effect with a couple of fingers. A lifetime of inhibiting aggression means a lifetime of aggressive energy stored and waiting for an outlet. Unless we come to terms with its very physical presence in our bodies, we may blow up at people near us, or induce our own ulcers and heart attacks. But aggression is a normal part of being human, and we can learn to work *with* its very powerful force, instead of against it.

THE USE OF ARMS

One of the most frequent complaints people bring to bodyworkers concerns the stiffness and aching they feel in their shoulders that sometimes travels up toward and into the neck. Disorders in the arms themselves are also common, such as the strain known as tennis elbow, which results from the stress of the tennis ball hitting the racquet when the elbow joint is held improperly.

Arms are used both for giving and receiving; when tension is present in the arms we not only have difficulty striking out on our own or expressing our feelings, but we also have difficulty simply reaching out for others. When you hold your arms back at all, that holding is likely to pervade all your activities.

If you walk around wherever you are right now, you will probably find that the swing of your arms begins somewhere behind the centerline of your body or, less likely, somewhat ahead of it. Wherever your arms begin to swing marks the line at which you are holding them—and your aggressive powers with them. If you choose to do so, you can work to release that holding pattern, freeing the energy associated with it, by imagining that your arms *can* simply hang from your shoulders, that you do not have to hold them in place any longer.

To begin to relieve the tension in your shoulder blades, armpits, elbows, wrists, and fingers, simply let your arms hang as you walk. Then, as you start to use your arms in picking up objects, pointing, touching, or

If you suffer from tennis elbow it is quite possible that you actually lead with your elbow rather than your wrist in executing your forearm strokes, with the result that your elbow is twisted in toward your body. If you lead with your wrist, with your elbow pointing out, the stress of the ball's impact on the racquet can be transferred to your whole torso, and the diminished impact on the elbow joint will be minor. If you pick up an imaginary tennis racquet now and execute a forearm stroke leading with the elbow, you will see that this movement results in the tennis ball hitting the racquet in such a way that it exerts torque on your elbow; the resulting strain is likely to produce the symptoms of tennis elbow sooner or later.

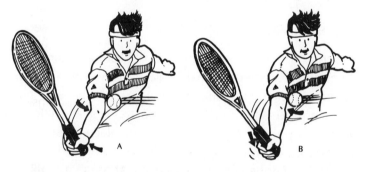

Figure 8-8. Forearm and wrist with racquet, hitting tennis ball (A) the usual way, which leads to tennis elbow, and (B) correctly.

reaching out to push something away or bring it toward you, move your arms without lifting your shoulders and without tensing your arm muscles any more than is necessary for the action you are performing.

Do you remember a time when you were angry at someone? Not at God or the elements or people in general or the circumstances of your life, but at a particular person? As you recall that person, that situation, and the feelings of that anger, notice where you begin to grow tense in your body. The energy of your feelings becomes apparent in the way you hold yourself, and you may especially become aware of your shoulders hardening and raising up, and of your upper arms growing stiff; or you may find your elbows pulling back, your forearms tightening, and your fists beginning to clench. The aggressive tension that originates in your arms may also read out into other areas of your body, including your neck and jaws, your feet, thighs, and buttocks, your abdomen, and your spine. Or it may not—but you have stored the tension of that anger somewhere in your body. We encourage you to be aware of the energy of aggression and how we all embody it. Only after we become aware of what aggression means to us can we hope to channel it productively.

THE HEALING TOUCH

Touch as the basis of healing is as old as the healing arts themselves. Other animals instinctively touch their wounds—lick them, nuzzle them, pat them—and humans are no different. It takes no training at all for a person to put her hands on a pain or place of physical discomfort; it is a wholly natural response of the body to the body. Sharing energies for healing through touch is a good portion of what the old-style family doctor used to accomplish with his bedside manner: touching, patting, and reassuring his patients; handling them. One of the great losses wrought by modern technological medicine is that medical schools have come to teach so little about this part of the doctor's art. Their concern with hygiene and sterile conditions—which are of vast value, to be sure, and which we do not wish to belittle—tend to discourage rather than encourage touch. As a result many otherwise excellent doctors have fallen out of touch with their patients.

The primary use of our arms in everyday life is to

accommodate our need to touch. Whether we reach out to hit or to embrace, we touch to make physical contact, and we touch to communicate. Numerous studies have demonstrated that contact through touch is a necessary aspect of any warm-blooded organism's healthy development. Without adequate touching, people (as well as other animals) become depressed, withdrawn, and hopeless. It is not too much to suggest that the proscription against our natural need to express ourselves through touch, as well as the scarcity of touch we experience as a result, constitute a major cause of mental, emotional, and physical dis-ease in our culture.

As we observed in Chapter 7, nearly every word in our language that addresses intelligence has to do with touch or the hands: We learn through manuals and handbooks about the subject at hand, we comprehend, grasp, handle, catch on; on the other hand, the aspect of touch that has to do with manipulation is concerned with having a handle on things so that they don't get out of hand. These sorts of phrases are not just handy means of expression: They constitute a metaphoric way for us to keep our fingers on the pulse of meaning throughout our socialization and education.

Touch is an automatic activity for babies, both as a means of learning about the world and as a way of satisfying inner needs. We never lose our need for touch even though the written and unwritten laws we live under demand that we displace that need onto objects that are often inappropriate and sometimes not even minimally satisfying. While the baby reaches out to grasp instinctively and feels free to touch anything that comes into its purview, our educational process seems designed to interrupt this natural inclination, training us rather to absorb information visually and cognitively, and leaving us with our hands empty for the experiences that teach us naturally.

John Naisbitt points out in his best-selling book, *Megatrends,* that the more a person is surrounded by high technology, the more she demands physical contact with other people. He says that although media specialists feared for a time that the popularity of television would obliterate the movies, in fact movie attendance has been on the rise in recent years—perhaps because you can be at a movie with many other people, but you watch television more or less alone. And even though more and more catalogue and electronic buying is available every year, the most frequented public space in America is the shopping center, which has become a social gathering place for people bereft of adequate touch.

When as adults we handle merchandise in stores or fondle our tools and toys as if they could love us back, we are repeating the infant's deep and primal need to touch. We do so because hands-on experience is the way people learn most naturally: Because, like other animals, we humans learn first and foremost through the body rather than through the mind.

Clients often bring their discomforts to bodyworkers after they have been unsatisfied by visits to their doctors, who may palpate their bodies a bit but rarely offer any healing, reassuring, soothing touch. Their recognition of the importance of touch is part of the reason Hellerwork practitioners, Rolfers, and other bodyworkers who perform structural integrations are quite expressly adept at these kinds of healing arts. They have been trained through the hands-on, whole-body experience of their subject, not through a predominantly intellectual meandering through their field of inquiry. Whether manipulation and touch cure the ailments they address is an unanswerable question: Each situation is unique. But they do very often eliminate pain and its accompanying stress, setting up conditions under which the body is most likely to heal itself. It is no surprise, then, that an increasing number of people are visiting masseurs and bodyworkers of all kinds these days, seeking the touching experience that is missing from their lives.

Just as we learn most rapidly through the body, so the fastest, most natural communication takes place through touch. The body provides a link that allows a great deal of nonverbal, noncognitive, nonrational, analogical information to flow back and forth between people. You can obtain such information by exploring any object through your sense of touch: a sculpture, your lover, your own body, or even this book, for example.

Close your eyes and touch something with your hands. Run it across your face, your forearms, any part

of your body. You can come to know the scope of its dimensions—texture, size, temperature, hardness or softness—through touch in ways that your cognitive and visual abilities can never provide. This is not to say touch is the only way or even the better way, always, to learn about something. But touch is a primary avenue of learning that is much neglected in our times, and you cannot touch until you can reach out and give, nor be touched until you can be reached and are ready to receive.

CONTROL AND SURRENDER | 9

THE PELVIC FLOOR

We now pass from our consideration of the body's superficial musculature to that of its deeper structures. We have already described the superficial muscles as the body's sleeve: those structures, relatively visible under the skin, that are involved principally in gross movement. Inside this sleeve is a central column, or tower, consisting of the vertebral column and its associated muscles, which support the body's whole structure and carry its weight, and which are also concerned with fine movement. This tower is the body's core, and it is to the lowest part of the core—the pelvic floor—that we turn our attentions in this chapter.

After three sessions of Hellerwork the sleeve usually looks better aligned and balanced than it was previously; it may be as much as an inch or more longer because its compressions have literally been stretched out. The body as a whole remains short down its center, however, pinched through the middle like an apple. From top to

Can you imagine a football player dancing ballet, or a ballet dancer playing football? Both are possible, of course, but the images seem incongruous to us because our bodies recognize that neither athlete's training is conducive to the movements of the other's profession. Although there is some overlap, for the most part these different kinds of performers train different muscles for different tasks: the football player his extrinsic mus-

153

cles and the ballet dancer his intrinsic ones. To get a sense for yourself of the difference between using your large sleeve muscles and using your small core ones, simply pick up a paperclip or a pencil from a table, and then try to pick up a stuffed couch. Even if you could pick up the small object with the muscles you employed to move the large one, you would feel like the Hulk. And if you had to pick up the couch with your fingertips? Impossible for even the strongest of men. Apart from Hellerwork and Rolfing, few disciplines pay any attention at all to the body core. The practice of yoga encourages movement from the core by its emphasis on lengthening the spine, and such martial arts as *tai chi* achieve core mobility by asking participants to execute movements in slow motion. This forces them to use the core muscles and the smaller intrinsic muscles of the body because the large extrinsic muscles are simply too large to perform a job of such delicacy.

bottom the intrinsic line between the flower and the stem —the core—is short relative to its extrinsic flesh.

The fourth through the seventh Hellerwork sessions, devoted to the deep muscles, will lengthen the core by relieving *its* compressions, so that core and sleeve can once again be in balance. But the new balance will be loose and fluid and long, rather than tight and rigid and short, allowing graceful movements to emanate from the physical and gravitational center of the body and move out through the whole physical structure.

The fourth Hellerwork session, whose theme and contents are reflected in this chapter, specifically addresses the dual needs of controlling ourselves in the world around us and surrendering to what is taking place in our lives. We first learn about, and later express, these seemingly conflicting concerns primarily through the musculature of the lower pelvis, and through the three important body functions centered there: urination, defecation, and sex. While these functions are all controlled by the muscles of the pelvic floor, they are actually accomplished through *surrendering* that control. When control is surrendered, the structures of the pelvic floor and inner thigh are at ease, and the pelvic floor supports the abdominal contents and can relax or contract as the occasion demands. Once we let go of tensions in this part of the body we discover how much these tensions have obscured the pleasures we can take in the most ordinary activities of the body.

UPTIGHT: TENSIONS IN THE PELVIC FLOOR

Anatomically, the core may be understood as the musculature around the spine, inside the pelvis, and in the flesh of the inner thigh—this last anomalous because it is available at the body's surface simply as a result of our having two legs. It is as if below the pelvis a single column supporting the core's foundation has been vertically bi-sected. If you can imagine people as mermaids or as the fish we are supposed to have evolved from, you see immediately that the insides of the thighs belong tucked away deep within the body where they could be well protected. For many people the inner thighs still feel highly vulnerable, and may be the seat of great tension —particularly tension associated with the other nearby deep structures of the pelvic floor such as the genitals and buttocks.

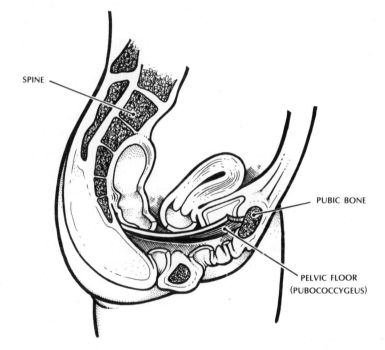

SPINE

PUBIC BONE

PELVIC FLOOR
(PUBOCOCCYGEUS)

Figure 9-1. The pelvic floor is made up of a hammocklike muscle known as the *pubococcygeus,* which supports all the organs that rest within the pelvis. Its fibers run mostly from front to back, from the pubic bone to the coccyx, reaching around the genitals and the anus and attaching to the inside of the pelvis, very near where the muscles of the inner thigh attach. The fascia covering the inner thigh muscles extends over the bone and becomes the fascia that covers the pelvic floor. There is, then, an intimate physical relationship among all these muscles that can be read in a psychological profile of a person as well as in the way she holds and uses her body. Another name for the pubococcygeus is the *levator ani:* the elevator of the anus.

155

Indeed, tension in the pelvic area is all but universal: Almost no one is entirely free from it, because in nearly all societies it appears with the onset of toilet training, when we are all asked for our first measure of self-control.

Up until about twenty-four months of age, the baby's anal sphincter is not yet operative, which means that the bowel is an open tube. Everything that comes down comes out, and there isn't much the baby can do about it. As time passes and the muscle is worked, it gains strength and is ready to do its job. But before this happens most parents start to exert pressure on the baby to hold its shit together, and most babies respond by doing the best they can, which is to tighten all the other muscles they can control around the sphincter. These muscles, of course, are those of the buttocks and inner thighs, and their early constriction makes them ready repositories of holding and tension forever after. As more and more control is demanded of the child—to control its bowels, its voice, its temper—the issue of control becomes further generalized, so that a person who has self-control is not supposed to leak any liquids or gases from his body; neither to shit, piss, fuck, barf, retch, cry, sweat, drool, run at the nose, fart, hiccough, burp, belch, or bleed—either physically or emotionally or linguistically—except at selected times and never in public.

This can be done! Given certain containers, including specified times and spaces into which organized and controlled discharge is permissible, such heroic control has proved possible. The cost, however, is huge. Physical and psychological tension is expressed in patterns of structural holding and tightness throughout the body, particularly around the area where it all began: the buttocks, inner thighs, and lower body core. This holding is one reason we call people who possess overabundant control *uptight* or *tight-assed:* The phrases identify the direction in which their pelvic floors are tilted and held.

Client: I was a bed wetter as a child, and during the session on control and surrender I became intensely aware that I had been holding onto my pelvic floor since I was three or four out of a fear that if I didn't do that I would wet myself again. I was finally able to loosen up, and in some unexpected way I found it took no work at all to not wet my pants.

156

While simple tension in the inner thigh and lower pelvic area makes it difficult even to spread one's legs, greater and more chronic tensions can cause the muscles in these parts of the body to pull on bones and muscles elsewhere, contributing to Charley horses and lower back strains, as well as constipation, hemorrhoids, distended

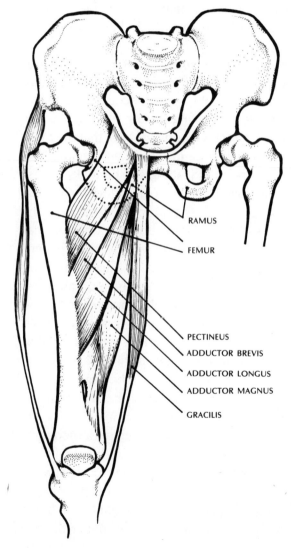

RAMUS

FEMUR

PECTINEUS

ADDUCTOR BREVIS

ADDUCTOR LONGUS

ADDUCTOR MAGNUS

GRACILIS

Figure 9-2. The muscles of the inner thigh are intimately connected with the pelvis and the pelvic floor.

157

Joseph: A couple of years before I was Rolfed I developed hemorrhoids. I had no idea why, or even what they were, really, and in retrospect I can see I was not very curious to find out or to do much about them. I was only dimly aware of them, and I wasn't especially eager to dwell on them. After all, if I went to a doctor I would have the embarrassment of dealing with a private part of my anatomy. Who wanted to have anybody looking up my asshole? So the hemorrhoids persisted. It wasn't until after my fourth session that I began to experience intense itching in the hemorrhoids, and over the next few weeks they shrank, dissolved, and disappeared, never to return.

colons and bladders, and a variety of urinary, colonic, and sexual dysfunctions.

One of the ways in which we civilized Westerners abuse the musculature of the pelvic floor is with the marvelous modern invention called the toilet. Obviously, this fixture is a great convenience, and so it is not the notion of the toilet itself that needs to be called to account, but rather its design, which does not suit its function very successfully.

In his twenty-year study, *The Bathroom,* Alexander Kira went to great lengths to demonstrate that sitting on a chair of normal height is an ineffective way to support the body while defecating. Kira's study bears out the experiences of structural bodyworkers, that the most natural and efficient posture for accomplishing this function is the squat. First, in squatting the buttocks are spread apart in a way that makes the pelvic floor the lowest part of the body's anatomy, except for the feet. Since there is no longer any cleavage at the buttocks, the anus can cut off feces cleanly and efficiently without toilet paper. Second, and more important, squatting exerts pressure on the anal sphincter. This pressure is important because normally peristalsis, the muscular contraction that pushes food along the digestive tract, travels down the intestines and stops at the rectum. Squatting initiates a reflex that allows peristalsis to continue on through the rectum to the anus. The familiar feeling of "having to go" results from the rectum being filled up so that its contents exert the same kind of pressure on the anus that is readily achieved by squatting. When sitting on a modern toilet, where rectal peristalsis is not activated naturally, people often feel they have to do something—push, strain, exert effort—to accomplish what takes place quite easily in a squatting position where there is nothing to do but let go. In the same way, squatting also turns out to be the ideal posture for urination, allowing the bladder to empty thoroughly while requiring no work of any kind.

Sex is the other significant function that takes place through the pelvic floor. While we can't just lie around waiting for sex to happen to us, we need not, as most people do, make some stupendous effort to achieve sexual release.

Take a moment to consider your own assumptions about the work required in order to have an orgasm: In what ways do you strive to *make* it happen? Certainly the body exerts autonomous efforts to encourage sexual release, but in addition to the involuntary secretions and contractions of the various relevant glands and muscles themselves, some people clench and tighten their entire bodies, particularly their pelvic regions, as if driving themselves toward some difficult barrier. This kind of rigidity inhibits sexual release rather than enhancing it, because it opposes the experience of *letting go.* Having an orgasm is a function the body is obviously designed to perform; any extraneous effort only serves to get in the way. Sweating and straining will not necessarily prevent the experience of orgasm, but orgasm is likely to happen more completely and pleasurably as a result of *relaxing* the pelvic floor and *surrendering* to the activity, rather than trying to control it all.

Client: The whole rhythm of sex changed for me when I learned to let go and enjoy myself. I used to have a kind of hard-driving rhythm, a mounting speed and pressure and intensity of movement and effort toward achieving my orgasm. It felt like pedaling a bike uphill. When I discovered I didn't have to do all that work I could allow my body to move in its own more natural, easy, flowing rhythm. The intensity mounted of its own accord, which was a very big surprise to me. I had believed I had to make an effort to build up sexual energy, and it turned out sexual energy built up on its own simply as a result of sexual activity.

PLEASURE AND REALITY

When they occur naturally, elimination and sex are experienced as extremely pleasurable, if for no other reason than that they involve the building up, holding, and release of energy. That three of the most common swearwords in our language—shit, piss, and fuck—concern pleasurable natural body functions expressed through the

J, who loved nothing better than feeling the flow of water carrying her along, stood beside a river and saw a tree full of dates on the opposite bank. Since dates were her favorite fruit, she decided to cross the river to get some of them. She could get them by surrender, which would entail lying down on a convenient raft or log and floating downstream; she could get the dates by control, by vaulting into a power boat and zipping across the water directly for the tree; or she could get them by sailing over the river, tacking back and forth until she reached the far shore.

In the first case, unfortunately, she would have no guarantee that she would ever reach the date tree, and so she might not get the results she desired. In the second case, she would be fairly certain to get the dates but would have no satisfaction in the journey. In the third instance only could she anticipate both pleasure in her activity and pleasure in reaching her goal. All the choices are legitimate, but our culture has chosen —as have most of us—to reach for the dates, the results, without reference to our journey, the satisfaction. Cultural rebels have usually chosen either to get to more dates faster or to sacrifice the dates altogether in favor of the pleasant ride. To have both the dates and the journey is possible, but only by choosing balance.

pelvic floor gives us a sense of the suspicion with which our culture regards pleasure, and the way in which we have imposed the social need for control on our so-called baser natures. Repressing the sexual drive is a very common way of restraining pleasure, for instance, and it results in considerable unnecessary tension. Women tend to work their inner thigh muscles in order to hold their legs together and keep themselves from opening up; men may withdraw themselves through tipping their pelvises and straining their pelvic floors, holding their penises back.

Wilhelm Reich wrote about the way child-rearing is intended to teach young people to sublimate their desires for pleasure into socially productive results. Perhaps the way we bring up our children reflects the way we direct our collective energy: away from natural enjoyments of all sorts and toward such constructed satisfactions as getting ahead in our careers, earning more money than we need in order to buy material possessions and status-rich experiences, and achieving positions of social power. It seems we have been persuaded that working hard for the approbation of others and for what other people regard as the general good is a better way to pass our lives than pleasing ourselves. It is hardly any wonder, then, that we have threatened ourselves with mass destruction and even extinction, while whole nations starve, lonelyhearts' pleas fill the want ads, and divorce courts and psychotherapists' offices are crowded with people who do not know how to express their love for one another.

One difficulty many people have fulfilling their own core needs is that in our culture we pay little attention to the body's core compared with the concern we heap upon the sleeve. We strive both as individuals and as a society for superficial power and beauty at the expense of deep support, endurance, and grace. In our athletic exercise and training, for instance, we concentrate on the appearance and utility of the extrinsic muscles while paying almost no attention to the intrinsic ones. It was Ida Rolf's contention that this imbalance in training—preferring the sleeve's bulk and speed to the precision and ease that emanate from the core—is one reason modern professional athletes' abilities decay quickly: their primes are very brief, and most professional careers are finished at a relatively young age.

Another difficulty lies in the way we have traditionally assigned social roles to the sexes. Most Western males habitually assert themselves as tough on the outside—with hard sleeves—while hiding their tenderness inside, at their soft cores. Women are more likely to present themselves in just the opposite way: soft and gentle at the surface, with a hidden hardness at the core. But regardless of gender, whatever attitudes a person embodies will be as apparent on the street as they are on the bodyworker's table. Those whose soft cores reside beneath a hard sleeve both feel and appear to be living within the prison of their tensions. Rigid on the outside and often rather spineless deep down, they tend to perceive their limitations as externally imposed, and they seek to liberate themselves by *breaking out*. People whose soft sleeves encompass hard cores frequently seem to be buried in protective padding. Yielding on the outside and often stiff in the center, they generally perceive their limitations as internally imposed, and they seek liberation for themselves by breaking *in*.

One way to understand these differences is that the lives of people who would break out are more likely to be dominated by issues of control, while those who think of breaking in are more likely ruled by issues of surrender. From the perspective of Hellerwork, both are unbalanced and incomplete, although the two concepts, which may appear at first to be antagonistic, are easily revealed as complementary components in this book's ongoing theme of balance.

CONTROLLING SURRENDER
AND SURRENDERING CONTROL

Freeze! Stop! Don't do that! Don't touch! Children are unbounded energy expressing itself most often in motion, but the first and commonest exhortations they hear from their parents and other adults are intended to create boundaries for them and limit their movements. Although we teach children to control their energies in order to channel them, control is usually more important to adults. Consequently, we think of good children as controlled children (children who are still) and bad children as those who fidget all the time and will not submit to our wills. As control of movement becomes associated for a child with obedience to authority, so loss of control becomes associated for the learning child with submission to another's will. The lesson is learned throughout the body-mind and is especially apparent in rigidities of the lower core, and in rigid attitudes toward the pleasures that are centered there, both in childhood and in later life.

What do you think of when you think about losing control? For most people being out of control means expressing intensely those feelings they have withheld from other people and even, perhaps, from themselves. To them, relinquishing control may seem frightening, as if it is a first step on the road to chaos. Other people regard losing control as leading to incompetence in the world, and they fear being unable to care for themselves.

Maintaining control is sometimes thought to be the positive end of a polarity whose negative end is surrender, since in our civilization surrender is usually understood as what the enemy does after losing a war. But letting go of control is not the same as losing control, and surrender is not the same as submission. Surrender is a willing accommodation of ourselves to reality, as control is a matter of imposing our will on reality. Surrender is a

Arnold Kagel is a neurologist and gynecologist in Los Angeles who used to specialize in incontinence—the inability to hold one's urine—which is a difficulty particularly marked in women who have just given birth. As a physician, Kagel knew that the balloonlike bladder is subject to special strain right after childbirth, because the pubococcygeus is rendered slack by the stretching to which it is subjected during delivery. He realized that in some women the muscle does not reassert its strength as rapidly or thoroughly as it does in others, and that its weakness places an additional burden of pressure on the small muscle of the urethral sphincter. It is this pressure, he realized, that results in some new mothers' incontinence.

In order to correct and prevent the problem, Kagel developed a series of exercises for his patients that gave them practice contracting and releasing the muscles of the pelvic floor. The exercises proved phenomenally effective, and also provided the side benefits of vastly improving his patients' sexual experiences, even leading some previously nonorgasmic women to have orgasms. Pursuing his original work, Kagel found that sexual dysfunctions in women were frequently nourishing nonaction, equally as necessary as the nourishing action of control.

As each of us seeks to define and assert that in ourselves which is unique, so each of us also seeks the experience of letting go, losing ourself, and subsuming our individual focus in something larger: a goal, a cause, a profession, a relationship. In what parts of your life do you experience surrender? What about control? How does each experience nourish you?

If you have ever seen a really fine surfer riding a big wave along the face of an ocean shore, you have witnessed a master of the balance between control and surrender. In order to ride, the surfer must control his board while surrendering to the wave. If he surrenders to his board, or if he tries to control the wave, he will certainly have a hard job instead of an exhilarating ride, and will probably wipe out. But he cannot control the board and surrender to the wave as two separate actions, because they involve him in a continuous fluid balance. He surrenders to the great force in which he moves while controlling the means through which he meets it. Skiers, skaters, and bicyclers do the same thing—as we all do, less dramatically, when we walk.

Lie on your back on the floor and tense your body from your feet to your head. When you are thoroughly tightened, try to roll over. You should find you are too rigid to move. Next, relax your body completely from your feet to your head, and try to roll over once more. Again, you should find you cannot move, because if you are fully relaxed you'd have to lie on the floor like a blob of putty. Neither complete control nor complete surrender is a useful posture in the material world: Rather, it is the *balance* between them that allows us to accomplish anything, and balance results only from combining control and surrender. The balance of control and surrender is defined by simple resistance.

related to weaknesses in the pubococcygeus, but that the problem was rarely a matter of the muscle being too slack: instead, he found, most people's pelvic floors were weak because they were hypertense. His exercises worked in part because they taught women to *relax* their chronically tight pelvic floors. These exercises have dramatically improved the experience of sex in men as well as women. (For further information on Kagel's exercises, see Ronald Deutsch's book, *The Key to Feminine Response in Marriage*.)

Client: I was afraid that if I let go of the energy that was binding my anger I would simply lose control of everything and blow it completely. But when I actually did let go and felt the anger I found I could let go of my fear of losing control at the same time. I surrendered to the emotional energy and did not have to fly off the handle. I could channel the energy at last, which saved me from having to explode, or blow up at anyone.

Joseph: As a bodyworker I sometimes used to find myself struggling to achieve a desired result: No matter what I did I could feel my client's body resisting me, refusing to let go. Then I would start to feel anxious and uncertain, and I would exert increasing amounts of effort trying to control the body beneath my hands: trying, in a sense, to *force* it to release its tensions. Clearly, what I was doing was not working, but I had become unable to see what the problem was. Eventually I discovered that if at these times of uncertainty I tuned into my pelvic floor I would almost always find that I was holding it tight. And when I found that out I could let go of these muscles very directly. Immediately my client's body would relax and our work could proceed.

163

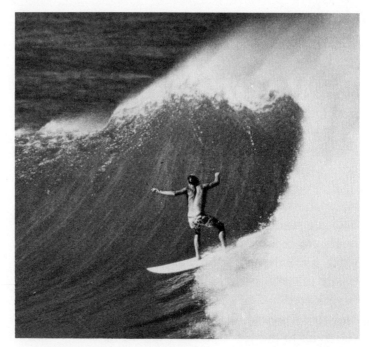

Figure 9-3. Surfer riding a wave in balance. Photo courtesy Jim Russi, copyright © 1986 *Surfer Magazine.*

THE IMPORTANCE OF RESISTANCE

The humble battery is a reservoir of electrical energy that must be made to flow between two poles in order to be productive. What is used to connect the battery's poles is called resistance. If you hook nothing between the poles you have zero resistance, and no current flows; if you hook up an insulator between the poles you have infinite resistance, and no current flows. In order for current to flow between the two terminals a finite amount of resistance is required.

In some ways electrical resistance is similar to tension in the physical body. When you eliminate all tension in the body, or when you eliminate all resistance with the battery, nothing flows, as you found out when you lay on the floor a couple of paragraphs ago. There is a necessary tension, a normal muscular tone, that helps us roll over, stand up, and otherwise live our physical lives. Up to a point we must increase that tension if we wish to increase our activities. For example, we need more resistance to move a piano than we do to pick up a coffee cup.

It is no less important not to use *too much* tension —not to use more than necessary, which is what most of us usually do. Pick up something small, such as a paper clip or a pencil or this book, and notice how tight even your large muscles become, how much of your body gets into gear to perform this little piece of work. Most people will feel their whole arm and shoulder grow taut; then the back tenses in conjunction with the belly muscles, the buttocks and legs tighten to support the other bodily tensions, perhaps the toes grasp for the ground below, the neck becomes a little stiff in bending forward, and so forth. Most of us actually exert our whole bodies picking up a cup and would have a hard time doing otherwise. In this regard we approach work mechanically, as if we were pieces of earth-moving equipment. All the same parts of the bulldozer move whether it is scraping up a few rocks or uprooting a massive tree stump. The alternative available to us, but not to the tractor, is to take the path of least resistance—to use the least amount of tension that will accomplish the job. This is the liquid, flowing, nonmechanical way. It is the way the human body is really designed to work.

One epitome of control is a high-powered car such as the Cadillac at the peak of its form: cruise control, climate control, power steering, power brakes, power windows, power antenna, power door-locks, power trunk lid, power heat, power air conditioning, power mirrors, power lights, power objects—not in Casteneda's sense—which you do not have to touch in order to be cushioned, supported, and cocooned in a way that enables you to minimize change in your environment.

Paradoxically, these technological marvels that isolate us from change simultaneously make us much more vulnerable to change than we were before we had them. We are highly adaptable creatures. The human organism responds to demand, just as its muscle tissue does, and the more demand there is to adapt, the greater becomes our ability to adapt. But when we have lived long enough in the Cadillac world we start to lose our adaptability. If our environment is perpetually warmed or cooled to a constant 68° to 70°F, the 60° beyond our doors feels really cold. The person who lives in a natural environment, however, may find any temperature between about 45°F and 80°F eminently comfortable. Most Americans have become more vulnerable to change than once we were, but most of us do not yet live in Cadillac worlds; we find temperatures comfortable between about 68° and 78°.

Gut Feelings, or Letting It All Hang Out

10

THE ABDOMEN AND THE GUTS

For most people, thinking about the guts brings on a queasy feeling of revulsion or disgust, as if the very subject were somehow unclean, unseemly, to be kept out of sight. We envision the guts in murky reds and fatty whites; they remind us of the lower depths of consciousness as well as the lower parts of the body, both of which are seen as bad, dirty, or at least somehow suspicious in this culture. The guts are the garbage disposal of the body, where stuff we don't really want to touch is flushed down out of sight, to be processed out of mind. When our feelings about the guts are not negative, it is generally because we are not thinking about them at all.

Our attitudes and dim awareness about the guts derive in part from all these organs being relatively primitive. They are related to the older nervous system that evolved in lower organisms to keep the innards working long before what we think of as the brain developed, and they function automatically. The guts do their job

Because of the usual human response to dark, warm, slimy things, French philosopher Jean-Paul Sartre considered nausea to be a condition of high existential anxiety. Consider your own reaction to steaming swamps and dank bogs, to stepping barefoot in thick mud, or lifting something squirming from a morass of viscous fluid. Do these images make you feel either anxious or nauseated?

Joseph: One frequent result of Heller-work is that even though we may not deal with diet explicitly and we do not actually enter the guts themselves except by pressing on the skin and muscle of the body wall, clients often report an increased awareness of their lower body functions, and then begin to experience specific hungers for particular foods—usually those that increase the body's ability to maintain its balance.

As people become aware of what their bodies really are and how they really operate, they seem to develop an understanding of their actual physical needs, which are often quite different from what they had previously thought.

whether or not we are aware of them, even though in our ignorance many of us make these organs work overtime by our relatively poor diet.

Guts is a term we usually use collectively to designate all the squishy contents of the abdominal and thoracic cavities, which are in fact one single cavity divided by the drumheadlike membrane known as the diaphragm. In the chest (the thorax), only the lungs are really part of the guts, while the abdomen contains most of the organs associated with three of the body's major internal systems: the stomach, intestines, liver, gall bladder, pancreas, and spleen from the digestive system; the colon and rectum—the lowest section of the intestines—and the kidneys and bladder from the eliminatory system; and the whole of the reproductive system.

What all these organs have in common, and what distinguishes them from that other major thoracic organ, the mesodermic heart, is that they are all composed primarily of endodermal tissue, and are primarily concerned with processing energy.

The most apparent energies processed in the guts are food, water, and air. The various organs break down the complex substances we ingest into simpler units our bodies can use as fuel, and they dispose of the rest. While it is clear that the guts process material energy, it is less obvious that they simultaneously process *immaterial* energy that might be construed as intuition, emotions, or "gut feelings," depending on your vantage.

GUT FEELINGS

No matter how the phenomenon is described, the guts process information about how we are responding here and now to the energies in our environment. Over the ages, the emotions have been a consistent source of wonder and mystery, but in the literatures of biology,

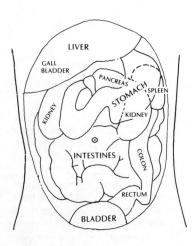

Figure 10-1. The guts.

physiology, and psychology there has been no thoroughly adequate explanation of their role in human nature. Most of us do not know where our emotions come from: They arise, often for no apparent reason, and sooner or later go away or change themselves into other emotions.

But from the body's point of view, the emotions we feel are the information our guts arrive at after processing the energy around us in a preconscious way. We moderns are so devoutly trained to believe that information can only arrive in the form of data to be processed in the brain that we forget how much information is offered by, to, and through our other faculties. We rarely think of a stomachache as information, for instance, and yet it is often the first and sometimes the only clue we have that something is amiss in our physiology. When you put your hand on a hot stove you withdraw it long before your thought of doing so tells you to, because you received some very clear sensational information.

We have lost many of our intuitive, gut feelings, but they can be regained. Do you remember the last time you walked into a room and had the sense or feeling that something was amiss? When asked to recall such situations, people generally remember their responses as a feeling, such as a tightening or tension, in the gut. It is only later, after the body has already processed the information those feelings indicate, that we start to look for rational clues to corroborate what our guts already know; but it is in such an experience of visceral instinct that our guts can best be seen serving their natural function of processing "immaterial" energy.

It is not yet clear whether in the course of our upbringing we are taught to shut down our ability to respond to the information our bodies provide, or whether we do so as a result of psychobiological programming that encourages humans to rely on their reason; but whether we

169

refuse to recognize our body's gift or are simply unable to take advantage of it completely, the talent is readily observable in children and much more rarely seen in adults. Somehow we seem to close off the expression of these feelings until we fail to recognize the feelings themselves.

It would be bad enough if we humans were simply denying ourselves the information our guts provide, because then we would merely be like people walking around with one eye closed pretending to themselves that they did not have two eyes. But the actuality is worse, because while we ignore it, neither the information nor our physiological response to it goes away. We literally carry in our bodies the feelings we fail to acknowledge about the truths we pretend not to know. We carry them in tense, tight abdomens that become hard walls with which we intend to keep our feelings at bay. We carry them in ulcers that we blame on worry, when the worry itself derives from our failure to acknowledge the feelings that trouble us.

Repressing these feelings also debilitates our confidence in ourselves and in our willingness to rely on what we know but pretend we do not know. When you are walking down a dark street at night and you suddenly experience fear for no apparent reason, it is possible that you are not just in the grip of paranoia or recalling the moment from your childhood when walking down a street at night evoked images of dragons and other ghouls, but that you are picking up an accurate signal of danger or hostility in your environment. In such a context fear is your friend.

The organism's response to perceived fear or fear that derives from something outside the body—walking down the street at night and seeing three shadowy figures starting to surround you—is a call to action and mobility:

to run away or prepare to defend yourself. Imagined fear, on the other hand, emanates from inside; therefore, the body has nothing to respond *to*—to fight or flee from—and so it tends to become immobile. But if you cannot or will not rely on your feelings, you have no way to assess whether something is really out to get you or whether you're just imagining it; and then you truly do not know what to do.

If you walk across your room right now, no one will think you are very courageous for doing so. But if we all know that there are twenty poisonous snakes on the floor your walk becomes very courageous indeed. People often think that courage means having no fear, whereas the truth is that there can be no courage without fear. Courage is action in the face of fear.

THE BUSINESS OF THE GUTS

As we have seen, thinking functions may be attributed to the ectoderm, action to the mesoderm, and feeling to the endoderm. It is a short step to realize that we live in a culture that does not want to know about the endoderm or its principal functions. We generally allow thinking, and we even encourage action; but feeling we consider weak, destructive, unstable, unimportant, and even dangerous, and we therefore disparage it if we recognize it at all.

In the business world, for example, we prize the cold, methodical worker who shuts out his feelings. We disapprove of bringing personal problems into the office, or making personal calls on the business phone. As a result, very few of us can be whole in our business environments. When our work environments reject large portions of ourselves, they become stressful and debilitating rather than supportive and nourishing. It is no wonder most people can hardly wait for five o'clock on Friday. How could they not want to leave as soon as possible so they can finally be themselves?

We have dehumanized business, behaving as if people are machines, robotlike elements of enterprise. This attitude has clearly alienated many people from the world of business who might otherwise be very happy and pro-

Joseph: My first office in San Francisco was a converted living environment in an old Victorian house, which provided a very familylike atmosphere. There was a kitchen where we all tended to gather and munch; people took showers in the bathroom and some would occasionally nap on their worktables. All in all the atmosphere was relaxed, and the office was much more like a home than your usual office. There wasn't the hurry to get out and go home that most people experience in more conventional work environments.

Bill: Some of the work I do as a counselor takes place in a residential facility—a house. While at work I frequently cruise through the living areas, nibble in the kitchen, may even take a shower. I find I usually go in to work a little early to chat with the other staff, and almost no counselors ever leave right on time when their shifts are over. We all stick around to chew the fat with one another, and both residents and counselors tend to hang out when nothing special has to be done.

Joseph: And "hang out" is the essential phrase, because people don't hang out in most business environments. Owners tend to hang out in their businesses because they own them and can feel at home in them. But from a manager's point of view hanging out is a waste of time. It's an unproductive, inefficient activity, something to be discouraged. But efficiency is not the only benchmark of business success. Success in business requires a full experience of both producing results and achieving satisfaction. While action leads to results, it is feeling that leads to satisfaction. Hanging out is what the guts do better than any other part of the body. Satisfaction comes through recognizing the guts.

ductive there. One of the ways we encourage this alienation is that we do not as a rule allow our business environments to support our guts. Very few office suites include kitchens, bedrooms, or full bathrooms, for instance.

Some business executives and managers have taken the Hellerwork series as a way to improve their efficiency and effectiveness. Those who were already in professional situations that were right for them generally accomplished their goal. As they relaxed their stressed bodies, they felt and looked looser and more youthful, ate healthier foods, and needed less sleep than they had before. Others, however, who had entered the world of business primarily because they thought they were supposed to, but who were actually not very comfortable there, decided by the end of the series that their real goal was to remove themselves from the stress-provoking environment in favor of finding satisfaction in some other arena.

This is not to say that any given individual should or should not work in the world of business, but that we all need balance in our lives. Since the guts are at the center of the body, they are fundamental to our ability to be in balance. The balanced body is able to process all the information it receives—physical, emotional, and intuitive, as well as cognitive—and finds the life circumstances that best support its need for balance, whether that means being an entrepreneur, bodyworker, teacher, cook, or anything else.

Not only does the balanced person find and maintain herself in the environment that is appropriate, she may find it increasingly difficult to feel fulfilled in environments that are not right for her. That is why wellbeing involves taking care of your guts. People rarely feel well when there is a turmoil in their guts, and guts in turmoil suggest imbalances that must be attended to, in order for the being to be well.

THE PSOAS IN ITS STRUCTURE

Many people who seek bodywork are mainly concerned that they have too much stomach: They think they need to reduce their potbellies or tighten their belts some other way. Many of them want to do sit-ups in the belief that they have weak abdominal muscles the sit-ups will strengthen. But their muscles are not usually the problem; they are tight already. Rather, it is the forward tilt of the pelvic bowl that forces the guts to spill from their appointed place. Although doing sit-ups will sometimes establish a new balance between the front and back of the abdominal wall, structurally sit-ups simply shorten the front muscles, making them as short and tight as the back ones, which have already been shortened by the pelvic tilt. This process of balancing shortness with shortness further compresses the core of the body and actually exacerbates the problem the person was trying to correct with sit-ups in the first place.

The pelvic bowl is a bowl indeed, and the shape of the container affects the workings of the container's contents. The organs of the guts are enclosed in a container of connective tissue composing the thoracic and abdominal walls. In working on the guts, the bodyworker is concerned with the front, side, and back muscles of the abdomen, as well as with the large group of muscles called the psoas (pronounced *So-as*), or the iliopsoas, located at the inside of the spine, or on what we might call the front of the back.

The cylindrical psoas—filet mignon, in beef—is one of the few large core muscles. It is unusual also in that, while most muscle groups move from one area of the body to another in stages—one muscle connecting torso to pelvis, another linking pelvis to legs, and so forth—the psoas passes directly from the spine through the pelvis to the legs. Centrally located as it is, the psoas is a muscle

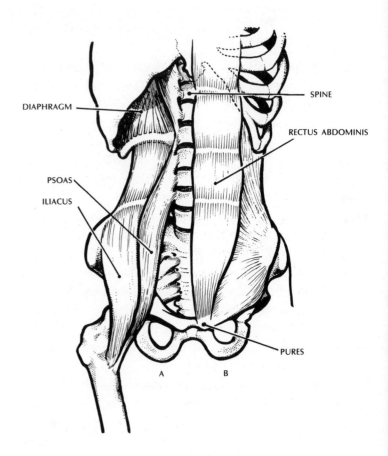

Figure 10-2. The muscles of the guts. (A): deep musculature; (B): surface musculature.

of considerable power; it accomplishes a great deal of work with relatively little effort.

Among its primary functions, the psoas acts as the main flexor of the hip joint, meaning that it should be involved in any movement in which you bend at the hips, whether by leaning, bending the trunk, or lifting the knees. However, if the pelvis is tipped forward, the functioning of the psoas is seriously impaired and it grows short and tight to compensate for its tension. This misalignment is very common. We usually describe it as swayback. It is a condition that requires the muscles on the front of the abdomen to do extra work to bend the trunk, and the muscles on the front of the thigh to do extra work to lift the legs. If you experience fatigue or pain at the front of your thigh when walking up hills or climbing stairs, a tight psoas is one likely cause of your distress.

When the psoas begins to grow short and tight, it pulls the rib cage down toward the pelvis, causing compression in the whole abdominal region. It is this compression, more than fat, that accounts for those bulges many people display above the crest of the ilium, which are known euphemistically as love handles. Rather than warning of impending obesity, love handles show that too much material is present for the allotted space to

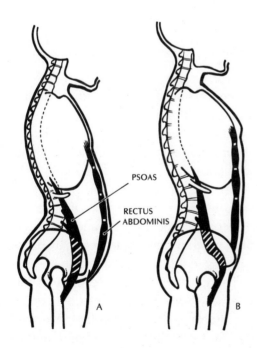

Figure 10-3. Relationship of the psoas and rectus abdominis. (A): Imbalanced and causing swayback due to a tight psoas; (B): Balanced.

accommodate, and warn of structural problems deeper in the body. This is the reason that when we elongate the psoas and the abdomen in the course of Hellerwork, love handles spread out and tend to diminish or to disappear altogether.

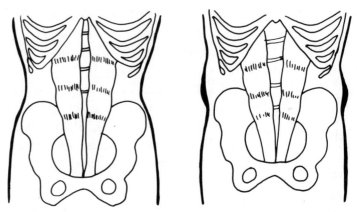

Figure 10-4. "Love handles" appear when the space between the rib cage and the pelvis is compressed. When pressure on the torso is released, the space increases and the love handles recede.

The compression that causes love handles also incites compression problems in the spine itself over the years, resulting in such ailments as lower back pain and sciatica. More immediately, it produces three kinds of physical debilities: First, breathing becomes restricted because the psoas is attached to the spine near the diaphragm, and tension on the former induces tension on the latter. Second, as the digestive and eliminatory organs are compressed, they become increasingly prone to spastic colon, colitis, constipation, diarrhea, and similar dysfunctions. Third, since a shortened psoas is functionally the same as a wholly shortened body core, it almost necessarily affects sexual functioning adversely.

The psoas is part of the musculature that moves the pelvis back and forth in the act of sex. When it is tight, that swaying motion is hard work; as a consequence,

Joseph: I was surprised to hear from a client of mine that after her fifth session she was able to give up her addiction to laxatives. Upon investigation I found that her condition is not uncommon: Many uptight people in our culture seem to need laxatives, which constitute the third-largest-selling group of over-the-counter medications sold in the United States after aspirin and cold remedies.

people whose psoases are tight become fatigued easily while making love. A second consequence of a tight psoas is that the sensations of sexual pleasure and orgasm are restricted to the genitals. On the other hand, when the whole body core is released, the psoas is activated automatically as well as intentionally, and the sex act becomes virtually effortless: The movement of the pelvis becomes something that seems to happen to you rather than something you have to do, sex becomes energizing rather than ennervating, and the sensations of pleasure and orgasm can be experienced throughout the lower part of the body and eventually throughout the entire body.

What has this got to do with you? You may not even have known you had a psoas until you started to read this chapter, and now here we are telling you all these horrific things about it. This is part of the problem: Whether the psoas is functioning well or not, people are mostly unaware of it; therefore the degree of control they can exercise over it is small.

A tight psoas is rarely an isolated problem. It is usually accompanied by tension in the rib cage and back, difficulty in breathing deeply, and other discomforts, because a tight psoas is virtually always part of a body that is tight all over. For this reason it is difficult to offer an exercise in a book that will release your psoas, but for starters, we can invite you to become aware of where the psoas is and how it functions.

Lie down on your back, on the floor or a hard bed, with your knees up so that your feet are just below your buttocks. Now, use the fingers of both hands to probe your abdomen about two inches to either side of your navel. Relax your abdominal wall as you let your fingers slowly move deeper into your belly. Holding your fingers as deep as you can without causing yourself much pain, gradually lift your knees until your feet are off the floor.

It is not our intention to suggest sex positions here, only to let you know how to arrange your body to make the exercise as easy and as fruitful as possible. Nonetheless, it will be worth your while to observe how you responded to the discussion of sex in the last chapter and in this one, even in a book about the human body. After the sexual revolution has come and gone, do we still have cultural injunctions against sex? Or do our proscriptive attitudes about sexual expressions reveal rather a broad distrust of the body altogether?

What was amazing about *The Hite Report,* published a few years ago, was that a large percentage of respondents expressed negative feelings about the whole sexual area of their bodies: Women felt their genitals were ugly, bad, unattractive, and a turn-off; men felt anxious about the size of their genitals and their ability to perform. People of both genders expressed attitudes of inadequacy, not trusting that their natural equipment was good enough.

If you think you are not adequate sexually, and if other cultural injunctions cut you off from the sources of your inspiration, prevent you from standing on your own two feet, keep you from reaching out for what you want and need, demand that you not leak from any of your orifices, and prompt you to feel revolted by the thought of your own intestines, as we have suggested is all too often true here in the midst of advanced Western civilization, how can your body possibly *not* be charged with the tensions, stresses, and anxieties you must be living with all the time? How can you make love with another person when you do not love yourself?

Joseph: Before I had bodywork I would have said I had no problems with sex at all. I was very active and

The muscle you feel tensing up against the back wall of your abdomen is the psoas.

If you want to take this exercise a bit farther, remain on your back and tilt your pelvis up toward the ceiling. With your hands on your abdomen, feel whether the wall of muscle tightens and shortens as you raise your pelvis or whether it releases and falls in. If it tightens, you probably use your front abdominal muscles habitually for abdominal lifting; if it releases, you probably use your psoas. If you find you are almost unable to raise your pelvis without tensing the front of your abdomen, you can be fairly sure you are not using your psoas optimally.

There is no way to fundamentally alter the condition of the psoas through reading this or any book, because effecting such a change is more a matter of rebalancing the entire body than it is of relaxing this single muscle. But if you practice moving your pelvis back and forth as loosely and as effortlessly as possible, without tightening your buttocks or the front of your abdominal wall, you will find as time goes on you are using your psoas more and more. Begin with a very small movement, and if you are willing to practice regularly, you can gradually increase your range. If you are so inclined, you might even pay attention to the way you make this kind of movement in the sex act and practice moving your pelvis as effortlessly as possible, starting with small movements, while making love. The sex act version of this exercise, incidentally, will be easiest to self-observe and practice when you are the partner on the bottom in the missionary position, or however else you can be lying on your back.

FREEING THE PELVIS

Repression in the abdominal area has negative repercussions in at least four of the body's major systems: respiration, digestion, reproduction, and elimination. But of course there is more. The solar plexus, located just below the sternum, is the second-largest plexus of nerves in the body after the brain. Even in our culture, where the concept of energy as we have discussed it in this book is not universally accepted, we recognize it as some kind of energy center; and since it embraces the heart, we have also accepted it by tradition as the seat of the emotions.

From the perspective of bodywork, emotional and physical systems are intricately intertwined. You cannot

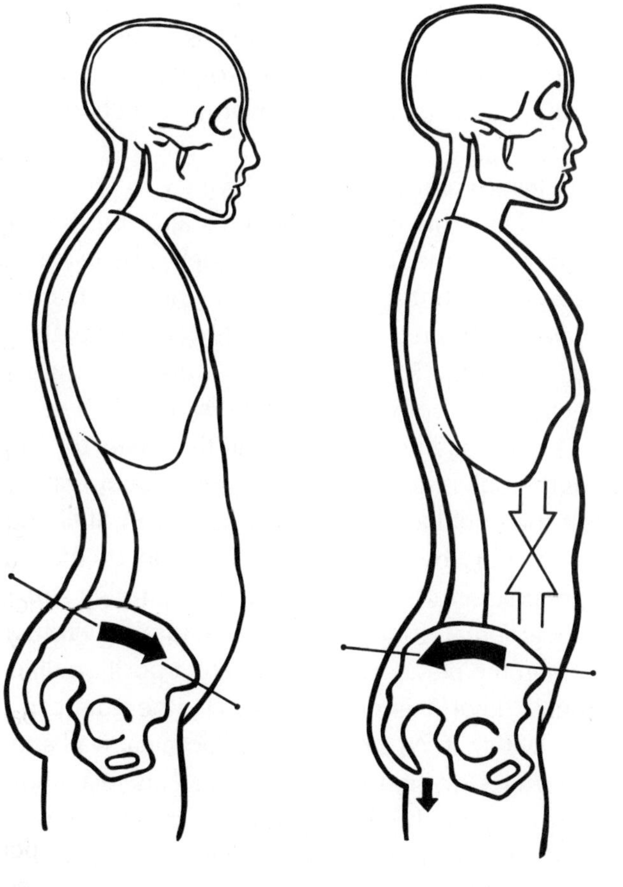

enjoyed sex a great deal. Yet with hindsight I can recall that moving my pelvis required effort I did not think of as effort, and the unnecessary work I was doing resulted in two symptoms I did not think of as symptoms at the time.

First, my lower back would get tired during sex and sometimes ache, and second, my energy would become depleted by the act so that after orgasm what I generally wanted to do was to roll over and go to sleep. The sensations of pleasure I experienced were also fairly well limited to the genital area.

Over the weeks and months that followed my session on the guts, my pelvis started to move on its own: My pelvic motions during sex were happening to me rather than happening as a result of something I was doing, and the whole act ceased to be tiring. My lower back no longer ached during sex, and after orgasm I would find myself energized rather than depleted. Finally, the feelings of pleasure that result from sex expanded throughout my pelvic area and eventually throughout my whole body. At that time I was simply delighted with what had happened to me, although today I understand that sensation travels better in loose tissue than in rigid tissue, as we have said several times in this book. My body became looser and the experience of sex became more fluid.

Figure 10-5. Pelvis tilted to spill the guts (L) and aligned with gravity (R).

even begin to get in touch with and openly express your emotions without letting go of physical tensions in the abdomen. In this regard, Wilhelm Reich, Alexander Lowen, Moshe Feldenkrais, Milton Trager, and just about everyone else concerned with the body as a functional structure are in complete agreement. It was Ida Rolf's unique contribution to freeing the energy restrained in the abdomen to realize that the guts are structurally supported in the bowl we call the pelvis, and that the position of the pelvis has a great deal to do with the state of tension or relaxation expressed in and by the guts. If your pelvis is tilted so that you are spilling your guts all the time, your muscles are always working to hold these sloshing contents in, and you never have a chance to be relaxed.

In Hellerwork, as in Rolfing, we try to mobilize the client's pelvis. This was also Reich's aim. But Reich attempted to free the function of the pelvis by using other functions of the body, such as having his clients breathe and move in directed ways to identify and break through their psychosomatic blocks. Reich's approach worked, but because the body is a unified system, not a series of isolated components, it took about five years for him to release the pelvis. Ida Rolf used to joke about that, since she felt she could accomplish the same sort of liberation in ten sessions by affecting the function of the pelvis through its structure. Affecting function through structure is a fundamental principle of all structural integration.

When the pelvis is held in an erect position, like the horizontal bowl it is designed to be, the guts can rest securely within it. As a result, the abdominal wall and the other muscles of the trunk can relax. This relaxation, in turn, allows the pelvis itself and the surrounding muscles to relax, and it increases the pelvis's overall mobility. Once the rigidity that impairs pelvic movement has been relieved, all twisting, rotational movements of the torso, such as those involved in walking, skiing, dancing, sex, golfing, or batting a baseball, have a wider latitude.

A LEG UP ON THE GUTS

Of all the activities enhanced by a mobile pelvis, walking is the most common, so let's take a walk now, just up and down the room.

Most people have the experience that their legs begin at the hip joint, and if you look at a skeleton it appears that in general this experience is correct. But if we take a muscular, rather than a skeletal, view of the legs, we arrive at a different picture.

Remember the last time you had chicken for dinner? If you take a chicken leg and pull it out from the chicken, the muscles do not separate at the hip joint. Rather, they

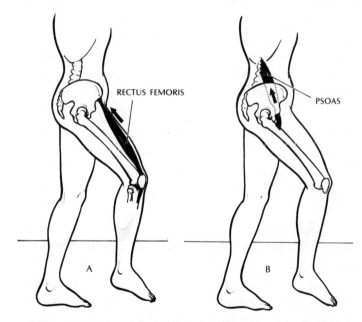

Figure 10-6. Walking from the thigh (A), and walking from the psoas (B).

181

separate at the highest point connected to the front of the spine, just below the rib cage at the level of the solar plexus. They separate, in other words, at the psoas. Muscularly that is where both human and chicken legs swing from.

If you would, place a thick telephone directory on the floor, or any object high enough to give you some elevation. Step up on your prop with one foot, and swing your other leg back and forth from the hip joint, feeling its movement in your leg and in the rest of your body.

Now imagine that you are swinging that same leg not from your hip but from your solar plexus, and notice that this time your whole lower body is involved, including your pelvis and your lower spine.

Next, step off your prop and walk up and down the room again, trying out the two different walking movements: first imagining that your leg moves from your hip joint, then imagining it moves from your solar plexus. You are likely to find that the second way results in a slight back-and-forth swing of the pelvis, spine, and sacrum (which is the lowest bone between the two hip bones). When you walk slowly from the solar plexus, the gentle undulation of your spine serves as a pump for all the fluids in your body, from the cerebrospinal fluid in your spinal cord to the various liquids resting in your pelvic bowl. The greater the degree of relaxation you impart to your walk, the greater the degree to which you encourage the all-around health of your body. In practicing this walk you might think of your pelvis as a bucket full of water, suspended by a handle at your solar plexus. If you hold the bucket rigidly, its contents will slosh out onto the ground; but if you let the bowl sway with the natural movement of your walk, both bucket and contents swing together and nothing is ever spilled.

When we speak of the guts we are discussing a body structure that is intrinsically fluid, and yet we have built

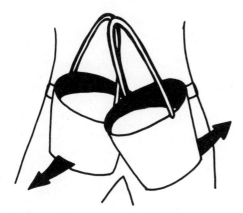

Figure 10-7. The pelvic bucket in walking.

ourselves a world that does not support fluidity of movement, fluidity of intelligence, or fluidity of any other kind. We hold our bellies tight, and our mythically macho heroes take pride in being able to withstand heavy punches to the gut without flinching. Our cultural attitudes are reflected in our bodies, particularly at the heart of the core, which is the guts. We have built a world of rigid structures, straight lines, flat planes, right angles, and hard materials, with hard rules enforced by hard-asses. The hard fact is that we tend to be too hard-core for our own good, and we are hard up for a bit of softening that will allow us to ease up, let go, and come to our senses with a better balanced perspective.

Before we examine the issues of balance and integration in terms of the body as we have come to know it so far, let's see how tension in the soft part of the body's core, the guts, appears from the perspective of that central mass we mentioned earlier, the central column of the core, the spine.

HOLDING BACK

11

THE BACK

Holding back is an expression we usually hear as a direction that means the opposite of going forward. Holding back is pulling back, stopping ourselves from progressing or expressing ourselves in any kind of forceful, powerful, authoritative way. But holding back also involves an action and a part of the body. To hold back in this sense is to put tension into the back. And indeed, experience shows that this is a common practice: In repressing inspiration, independence, aggression, spontaneity, sexual energy, and their emotions, people do hold enormous amounts of tension in the back, and especially in the central column of the body's core, the spine.

STRUCTURE

The representation of the ideal human spine is the tensegrity mast, which we discussed in the first part of this book: a structure the continuity of whose integrity is

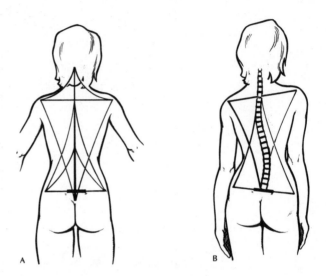

Figure 11-1. Ideally, the spine functions as a tensegrity mast on a balanced pelvic base (A); ordinarily, the mast is thrown out of alignment on an imbalanced pelvic base (B).

maintained through flexible, tensional members, and whose hard, compressional parts act as spacers to maintain that tension properly. In the spine, as elsewhere in the body, the bones are the spacers; the tensional members in this case are the muscles, tendons, ligaments, and fascia.

Ideally, the vertebrae/spacers are suspended in the tensional network between the discs. These discs act as shock absorbers, soaking up the impacts that compress the spine when you jump and hit the ground, descend in a fast elevator, or even walk. Under the best circumstances each disc closes and opens like a spring that is compressed and released, expressing the fluidity of the flexible mast that also makes rotational, bending, and oscillating motions.

Frequently, adults in our culture have spinal columns that are chronically contracted. This is because the discs are perpetually compressed by constant tension in the muscles and connective tissue and are only rarely and

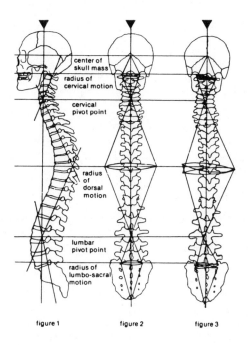

figure 1   figure 2   figure 3

Figure 11-2. Gravitational weight line.

incompletely released. If you think of the discs as springs, you can see that such perpetual pressure must eventually damage or destroy their original resiliency. Because the discs are composed of connective tissue, they are also subject to rigidification under these conditions. As a result, instead of maintaining their sprightly ability to bounce back and keep the spine mobile, the discs often contribute to its overall rigidity. When the compressed discs become effectively solid, the spine itself acts as a compressional rather than a tensegrity structure—like a great column of blocks stacked and glued one on top of another. The spine was not made for this kind of life, of course. Discs degenerate under such a load: They dry up and lose volume, further compressing the mast as the continuing degeneration and compression amplifies and feeds on itself.

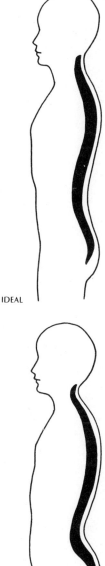

IDEAL

NORMAL

Figure 11-3. The ideal and the normal Western adult spines.

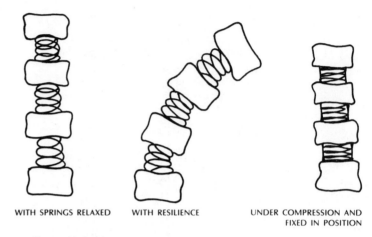

WITH SPRINGS RELAXED   WITH RESILIENCE   UNDER COMPRESSION AND
                                             FIXED IN POSITION

Figure 11-4. Discs as springs.

MUSCLES

As you might imagine, the spine's structure is deeply influenced by compression on the body's core. Compression, however, does not originate in the bones of the back; it shows up first in the muscles and connective tissues.

If you look at the back muscles structurally, you actually see a lot of leftover design from our species' quadrupedal history. The trapezius, the big diamond-shaped muscle that goes from the neck to the shoulder and on down to the middle of the back, doesn't make as much sense in an erect, two-legged animal as it would have made in a four-legged one, for example, where its multidirectional fibers could control the front-to-back motion of the front limbs.

If we adhere to evolutionary theory we can see where the stress of gravity once acted to contract the extensor muscles; even if you prefer some perspective on human life that is not evolutionary, you can see that the development of the individual human itself is a progression from four-legged to two-legged functioning: The baby begins life curled up in a more or less flexed position and gradually learns to straighten out and straighten up, its movements progressing from a four-legged creep to a two-legged stride. This development entails growing muscles in the back, largely after the muscles in the front of the body are already well formed. Because the back's extensor muscles are not yet developed, the very young infant lying on its stomach can neither lift its whole leg from the thigh nor lift its arms, back, or head.

BONES

Most of us mistakenly believe the skeleton is a rigid framework holding the body together, and we live as if that were true, literally holding on to our bones as if seeking stability. If you press in all around on your thigh you will probably feel a bonelike hardness at its center about three inches in diameter; yet the shaft of the thigh bone itself is only about one inch in diameter. The rest of the hardness you feel is *muscle,* squeezed rigid by the tension of clenching at the thigh bone—what we call holding. This holding is unnecessary: The bone will not run away from the muscles attached to it; and it is this holding that turns most adult Western bodies into compressional rather than tensegrity structures, with all the attendant stresses that implies.

It should be evident by now that a certain amount of holding is introduced to every body in the normal course of growing up and learning the rules of social living. Although some of these lessons may have been useful, we can assume that as adults we have already learned both the good ones and the bad, and we no longer need behave like children at our elementary lessons. Holding our breath, withholding our aggression and love, and all the other restraints and repressions contemporary flesh is heir to become destructive when they run counter to our body's very structure.

Grown up as we are, each of us repeats physical behavioral patterns that reinforce the habits we could not help but learn. For example, when we feel fear or anxiety or any other lack of stability, most of us reach automatically for the nearest stable object. We do this emotionally when we cling to other people we feel we can rely on for support in times of trouble, and we do the same thing in the flesh. If you are on a ship that suddenly rolls at sea you will probably grab for the guardrails because they appear to be stable; inside your body your muscles clutch at your bones the same way.

As any sailor knows, however, you would be far stabler on that ship if you simply rolled with its motion. You may recall from the preceding chapter that when you walk as if your pelvis were a bucket containing the liquid of your guts, letting it swing with your natural motion, your intestines float with you and do not have to be held in place; whereas if you hold the pelvic bucket rigid, the contents tend to move about more vigorously, and you are inclined to try to contain them by tightening your abdomen. In the same way, holding on to your skeleton makes your body rigid and unstable, while letting it loose allows you to maintain your balance even in life's rough seas.

PUTTING UP A GOOD FRONT

The corollary to holding back is putting up a good front. Like holding and instability, relaxation and balance are most apparent in the spine, which reflects virtually any tension anywhere in the body. If you clench both fists, then let them go, then tighten them again and let them go again, and repeat this process several times, you may notice that you cannot tighten your hands without also tightening the muscles that lead up to and surround your spine—just as if you clench and release your jaw a few times you will find that the back of your neck gets tight along with your jaw. When all these tensions and others from elsewhere in your body tighten up your tissues, they become part of holding back, holding *your* back, and holding *in* your back as well.

Back up, back off, back down, get off my back: get back means "move away." But for the body, getting back entails holding back, holding in, and tightening up by pulling physical and metaphysical energy in toward the core. According to Moshe Feldenkrais, negative emotions cause tension in the body's flexors—muscles that

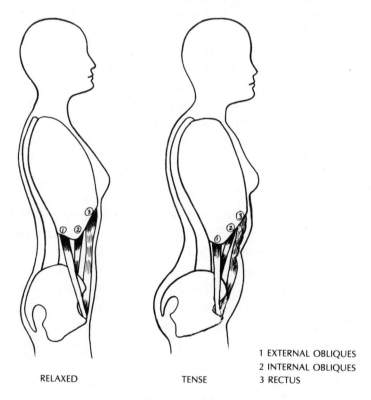

RELAXED	TENSE

1 EXTERNAL OBLIQUES
2 INTERNAL OBLIQUES
3 RECTUS

Figure 11-5. Musculature of front flexors.

bend parts of the body—particularly those in the front of the body. A natural response to anger, fear, or sorrow is to curl forward toward the fetal position, as if protecting the belly and guts. That curling demands tension in the flexors. If we do not express that tension through movement, we end up holding it in our abdomens; then in order to rebalance ourselves we have to counterbalance our tight front with an equal amount of tension in the back. The result of this sort of compensation is a balance of tension rather than a balance of relaxation, in which we compress ourselves together tighter and tighter.

Sit relatively straight in your chair and tighten all the front muscles of your chest and abdomen, allowing yourself to fall forward as those muscles demand. This is what your body is inclined to do any time you flex your torso. Now return to your upright posture and tighten all the same muscles, but this time do *not* allow yourself to collapse forward. You will notice that the only way you can avoid falling forward is by establishing a corresponding tension in your back, as a result of which you become very stiff and compress your body into the chair.

Bill: Before we did the session on the back, I was holding myself so rigidly that my spine felt more like a joint than a flexible mast. Lying on my stomach or sides on anything softer than the floor made me feel as if my body was being bent the wrong way: I felt as if I was going to snap. Consequently, I had been unable to sleep on my stomach or sides for several years. Now, I have freedom in the matter. I can sleep in any position.

OH, MY ACHING BACK

Some 75 million Americans suffer from back problems, according to a 1983 *Time* magazine article. Since children are not usually so disabled as to figure into such a count, the number implies that about one of every two adults in this country suffers from back pain in a meaningful way. There is no single cause for this virtual epidemic of back problems; rather, it is the combination of related factors that produces a slow erosion of the spine's structural integrity. When your back goes out, it seems like a sudden event: It seems that nothing warned you it was coming. What actually happened is that accumulated stress caused by many factors has overwhelmed the structure at its weakest place.

One reason people don't know what to do about back problems is that, both inside and behind us, they are invisible. There's no particular lump or bump we can see. As a result, a person who goes to the doctor with lumbar pain or sciatic nerve pain or disc pain usually gets treated at the site of the pain, even though the problem is almost always one of compression in the whole spinal structure.

We also don't see back problems before they erupt because few people are even aware of the factors in their lives that contribute to spinal compression. For instance, most people, men and women alike, wear heels on their shoes. Heels refer all weight to the forward part of the body, so that we are, in effect, standing on an inclined plane. We compensate for this unnatural posture by leaning our chests back, compressing the bones in our lower backs.

One possible, generally unpredictable result of a spinal blow-out is damage to or a disorder of the nerves. When a nerve is damaged, the parts of the body it controls are also debilitated. If the nerve leads to the leg or spleen, for example, pain or damage to the nerve in the spinal column may also cause pain to the leg or spleen. Another possible result is damage to the spine itself, such as degenerative disc disease. *Herniated* discs have gotten so badly squeezed they have been pushed through the weakened disc wall; *slipped* discs have been effectively squeezed out from between vertebrae.

The common medical solution to spinal ailments is spinal fusion, in which a wedge of bone is placed between two vertebrae to keep them apart so that they do not compress the nerve or the disc any more than they have already done. Sometimes traction is employed to decompress the spine. This is effective but inefficient, partly because the process is slow and partly because the client is entirely passive: In a sense he has no experience of having had anything to do with his cure, and he has not learned anything useful in his body that will keep his

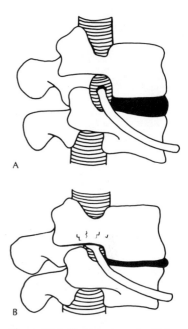

A

B

Figure 11-6. The hole through which the nerve emerges is made up of two halves, one belonging to the upper and one to the lower vertebra. The body is designed so that the spinal cord will pass through the middle of the vertebrae, with nerves branching out from the cord through dutch-door holes between them (A). As the vertebrae compress, the hole grows smaller and pinches the nerves (B). The pinch is exaggerated through rotation and bending movements, and thereby affects the nervous system.

problem from recurring. Certain exercises can slowly decompress the spine, but people usually do them so strenuously that they tighten their skeletal muscles even more, and no decompression results. Kundalini and Iyengar yogas are inherently rigorous, but integral and hatha

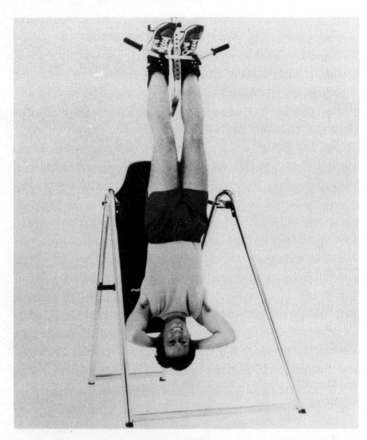

Figure 11-7. Some years ago, a Los Angeles man named Robert Martin started building Gravity Boots and a Gravity Guiding System, for hanging upside down. His theory was that hanging and brachiating are normal primate activities that we humans don't have much chance to do, and that these activities help to decompress both the superficial (hanging) and the core (brachiating) muscles. He found that one side effect of his product was to make its users longer—that is, taller. He developed as a clientele people who wanted to join the police and fire-fighting forces but were slightly too short to meet those departments' minimum height requirements. By following Martin's hanging program for three months, they could gain about a half-inch in height, which was sufficient for many of them to pass into the uniformed ranks.

yogas emphasize lengthening the spine with ease rather than effort, over the course of long and fairly dedicated practice. Hanging upside down can also relieve pressure on the discs; this is not a very sophisticated approach, but it is certainly more creative than the better-known options.

Chiropractors and osteopaths specialize in problems of the spine. But while their work is valid and valuable, they usually treat *only* the spine. Thus it is only a partial solution to a problem that affects the whole body.

Structural bodywork increases the fluidity of rigid tissue and restores tensegrity to the spine, at the same time realigning it so that the weight it bears is properly distributed. The success of this very simple approach to alleviating spinal decompression and helping to maintain a loose structure indicates that the whole collapse of the central mast of the body is not as inevitable as people have usually thought, and that it is reversible.

PHYSICAL EDUCATION

We have observed before that to a great extent our educational programs are committed to limiting, channeling, and imposing restraints on children's boundless energy. Of course, this is one way of teaching them to hold themselves back. Restrictions and prohibitions command the child to pull in his energy, which literally entails tightening up toward his center around his spine. The process of learning to hold back is accelerated when he is forced to sit still for six or eight hours a day in school—an utterly unnatural occupation for a youngster, justified only by the extreme position that, since sitting still is what the child will do when he grows up, he might as well begin learning early to be tight, tense, restrained, and immobile.

Immobilizing the child is part and parcel of teaching him to obey arbitrary authority and to take orders without question, stifling his creativity by breaking the back of his

Joseph: When I train Hellerwork practitioners, at one point I ask everyone to pretend to be a good boy or girl for a couple of minutes. Immediately people grow quiet and restricted. They contract, stop making contact with one another, stop looking at each other. Then I ask them all to pretend to be bad, and right away they get raucous and playful, make noise, move around, make contact with each other, and have fun. It would appear that when we teach our children to be good we are not teaching them anything about morals or ethics, but only about staying out of trouble. When you were a child you never quite knew what trouble was made of, but you did know you didn't want to be in it, and that is what "good" came to mean. The easiest way not to make trouble, of course, is not to do anything: Back up, back off, back down, get back.

initiative. We have grown so intent on learning as an intellectual activity that we have pushed into the background our awareness that learning takes place first and foremost through the body.

But the body does not forget, and simply in physical terms the cost of all this restriction is staggering. In later life it leads directly to sprained and strained muscles and ligaments, arthritic joints, hemorrhoids, prostatitis, ulcers, colitis, spastic colon, sciatica, pinched nerves, disc problems, temporomandibular joint dysfunction, headaches, vision difficulties, and more.

We have developed the belief in this century that stress and anxiety are psychological conditions located in the mind, which we somehow assume is situated in the brain. But wherever they may begin, anxiety and stress result in, are part of, and occur together with *physical* tension and structural imbalances.

People who are not concerned with the body in a systematic way might not see the relationships among these issues, but even research with rats affirms that behavior is intimately associated with structure. When we subject laboratory animals to anxiety, they develop sores and nervous tics, lose weight, lose their hair, teeth, and tails, and generally start to fall apart.

So it is too with human animals in the laboratory of our everyday world. Though we don't lose our tails, it is commonly observed that people under stress similarly fall apart: We lose our hair and teeth, we gain or lose weight, we grow jittery and anxious or sullen and withdrawn.

All in all, we can ill afford the behavioral cost of holding back. Individually, as we have been seeing, we spend a great deal of effort for little satisfaction and a lot of pain. Societally, we pay the price of creeping mediocrity: All around us people are holding back, failing or refusing to do their best. They do not contribute their creativity because there is no room for innovation or inspiration in most of our work environments or social

196

structures. They do not contribute their thoughts and ideas because they get no support to stand up for themselves; they do not contribute their feelings because when they do they are seen as weak. People hold back their power, initiative, and self-discipline in their jobs, their relationships, their personal growth, their performances everywhere, and we are all worse off for it. Holding back has become the norm. As a result, excellence, which is often just a matter of giving one's all, has become truly exceptional, as if it were a hard thing to provide.

Somehow we have become a culture that sees itself as needing to be inflicted on the individual rather than supporting him in achieving his best. We work hard to prevent people from doing wrong, or bad, or poorly, or whatever we deem to be outside their—that is, our collective—best interests. In effect, we make it difficult for people to give their all.

All these problems may make it seem that we back off from excellence because it is hard to achieve and because it is a hard taskmaster once it is reached. But excellence and ease *can* coexist; in fact, they exist together far more readily than do excellence and effort. It is easier to be excellent by being naturally expressive than it is by making the enormous effort required to hold back. Every book on anatomy is full of examples documenting our inability to build machines that are as reliable as our natural organs. We cannot begin to approximate artificially the range of situations to which human beings can adapt with ease. Ultimately, what all our holding back costs us is our excellence, both as individuals and as a society. We have been following both a personal and a cultural notion—mistaken in both instances—that excellence arises through rigidity, when in fact it is possible, almost always, only through fluidity. To a discernible degree, that notion is centered not in the core of our body structures, but in our heads.

LOSING YOUR HEAD | 12

THE HEAD, NECK, AND FACE

The head is the top of the body's core, and it is the seat of reason according to most of Western civilization. To lose your head, then, is to free this final portion of your body's anatomy from muscular rigidities, and simultaneously to take a step toward freeing yourself from rigid patterns of thought and belief.

THE HEAD AS THE TOP OF THE PHYSICAL CORE

Whenever you move, whether you are standing, walking, or riding in a car, your head will not fall off your neck; it does not need to be held in place with anything more than normal muscle tone. Ideally, your head would bob about pretty freely, a bit like the little spring-necked doggies some people place in the back windows of their cars. You would have a free-floating, light head.

Most of us, however, hold on to our heads as if we had to restrain them. At the movies, for instance, we hold

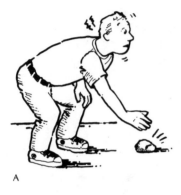

A

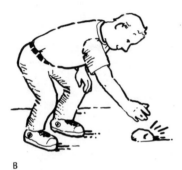

B

Figure 12-1. Neck hold (A); Neck released (B).

our heads rigid while looking at the screen; while driving we maintain pressure on our necks and shoulders as we grip the steering wheel or gear shift; and when talking to other people we usually hold our heads in some sort of rigid posture that reflects both our tension and our attitude toward our conversation partner: respect, subservience, eagerness, reluctance, and so forth.

Wherever you are sitting now, draw your chair back so you can bend down and pick up an imaginary piece of lint at your feet. The moment your fingers touch the floor, stop. Stay in this position for a few seconds, and notice what you are doing with your head. With your eyes directed straight out, are you looking at the bottom of your chair? At the floor beneath you? Or some place in between? Most likely, you are holding your neck and head up to some degree, as if you have to face the floor to pick up the piece of lint. If you have any doubts about your position, relax your neck muscles entirely now, and let your head drop forward as far as it wants to go, without pushing it. You will probably find it falls several inches. Leaving your head down as it has fallen, return to a sitting position, and notice that as you do so the released weight of your head can actually lengthen your spine whenever you make bending movements.

Return to the bent-over position in which you are about to pick up imaginary lint and hold your head up again the way that was natural for you to do just a couple of minutes ago. This is probably the way you hold your head most of the time. Maintain that position for half a minute if you can, and you will probably be able to feel your entire neck and shoulder area compressing, tightening, and shortening with the tension you have habitually carried in those muscles. Since your adult human head weighs some twelve to fifteen pounds, its muscles and those of your neck are currently exerting enough tension to hold up a bowling ball at an awkward angle—something you probably cannot do with your outstretched arm for more than a minute or two. But once you have released your head, those same twelve to fifteen pounds can help relax and lengthen your spine in bending movements, rather than compressing it. For example, let go of your head once more and see if you can feel the weight of your head literally stretching these very same muscles. Now, letting your head continue to hang down, return to a sitting position and feel as you do so that the weight of your head continues to stretch out your spine. This process of losing your head can accompany any movement at all.

THE HEAD AS SOCIAL CONTROL TOWER

In our society we have accepted logic and reason as the correct modes of apprehending to such a great degree that one of the worst things you can say about another person is that she is irrational, whereas rational is one definition of sane in most dictionaries. Sometimes it seems that in our extreme pride we believe life itself follows the rules of human logic—although, poised as we are at the brinks of chemical, biological, and nuclear catastrophe, mounting evidence might suggest to even the most rational mind the possibility that we are wrong, and that, although we like to think of our species as the rational animal, we seem to be the one creature on Earth that does the most consistently irrational things.

The notion that everything can and should be organized according to reason is a basic principle of most Western societies. This view is promulgated by people who believe that the physical aspects of being human are less important than the mental or emotional ones, and who seek to help us rise above the beastly part of our nature. Accepting that our fundamental unity can somehow be so split, they attribute what are supposed to be our good qualities—those our culture deems desirable

Lose your mind and come to your senses.
—Fritz Perls

It was Carl Jung's contention that one purpose of unconscious productions such as dreams and art is to provide balance for the exercises of the conscious mind. In this context it may be telling that America's major entertainment for the past decade has been fantasy films ranging from the space fictions of *Star Trek* and *Star Wars* to the larger-than-life adventures of Superman and Indiana Jones.

The other side of the coin is that the body expresses what Jung might have regarded as the shadow side of our collective rational life in particularly 20th-century illnesses such as cancer, a highly *irrational* disease based in uncontrolled growth of mutant cells.

because they are least animal—to the highest and most visible place, the head, and our worst aspects—those seen as undesirable because they are most animal—to the pelvis, the lowest, most hidden end of the physical pole. We might say, then, that in our culture the head represents the reasonable, and the pelvis the passionate, sides of our natures. Passion in this regard includes not merely instincts and emotions, but also an openness to the magical, mysterious, and unexplained. One result of our passion for logic is that for the most part we have given up or lost the innate sense of wonder and mystery about life we had as children, and substituted for it the illusion that sooner or later we will be able to explain the whole universe rationally.

In some ways these distinctions between the rational and the passionate seem quite arbitrary, but in others they appear to indicate something true about human nature. Certain occupations, for instance, *are* more intellectual, more up in the head, than others, and they seem to foster or attract people with particular body types and postures. It is a rare boxer or football player whose head is not tucked in tightly to his torso, where it can be protected. But consider the seemingly disproportionate number of attorneys whose necks stretch forward and who lead with their heads. Is this a result of hunching over papers in the law library? Is it a way to reach out with their words? Is it a way to put their noses into other people's business? By reaching forward with their heads they are able to bring their faces closer to other people, which may make them more persuasive when they have to face off with others.

It may be that our headstrong culture is reflected in the degree of dis-ease we have centered in the head. Not only psychological difficulties, which, as we have been observing throughout this book, find expression through other parts of the body as much as they do through the

202

head, but also through such physical ailments as headaches, temporomandibular joint dysfunctions, and vision problems that are prevalent today. Close to half the adult population of this country wears some form of corrective lens; cold and headache medications such as aspirin are the largest-selling nonprescription drugs in America; and TMJ disorders are commonly seen by dentists in this country, where we consume more chewing gum than any other nation in the world. All three of these classes of discomfort derive from tension in the head, specifically in the suboccipital muscles—those muscles in the back of the neck that attach to the back of the skull and become tense when the neck leans forward.

THE NECK

In the seventh Hellerwork session we try to help people become aware of how they hold their heads, which is usually related to tension in the neck and head muscles. When the client is lying on his back on the table, the practitioner rocks the head back and forth and lifts it gently; tension manifests as a general sense of resistance to these attempts.

You might take a moment now to lie on your back, on the floor or a firm bed, and place one hand beneath your skull where it comes to rest on the flat surface so that the occiput fits in the palm of your hand. Using only your fingertips as leverage, lift one side of your head slightly, then let your head roll back, pushing your fingers down. Do this a few times to get a sense of the rigidity and holding in your own neck and head that actually prevent a full, flowing roll from taking place.

When you lie on your back with your knees up you will also notice that your neck is chronically pushed forward, so that it is almost impossible for your neck to lie flat on the floor or bed. Instead, it will form a kind of

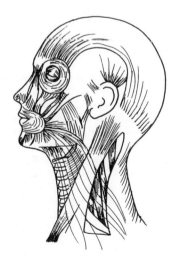

Figure 12-2. Musculature of neck and head, side view.

203

Joseph: I have a friend who used to sport a beard, and who, after many years, decided to shave it. When he did so I saw that part of his motivation for wearing the beard in the first place was that he had quite a small, recessed chin that looked very much out of proportion to the rest of his face. The beard had made it look more balanced and proportionate. Confronted with this feature after he shaved, he met with an orthodontist who suggested orthodontic surgery to extend his jaw forward. Before going under the knife, my friend asked me if we could do anything about his chin through bodywork. We spent several sessions balancing his body, at the end of which he felt his appearance was sufficiently different that he was no longer interested in surgery.

Joseph: Before I was Rolfed I thought my body was a moving pedestal for carrying my head around. Several science fiction films have portrayed an idealized brain floating around in some kind of vat, moved around when necessary by acolytes and addressed directly by people who wanted information from it. That is how I felt about myself. What was important about me was all up there. Once my head was realigned, however, I felt as if it were floating on top of my neck rather than weighing the rest of my body down: as if a weight had been lifted off my shoulders. I felt more connection between my body and my mind as a whole than I ever had before.

bridge beneath which you can insert two or three fingers. The neck should not be straight when you are standing, because the spine does have some natural curvature, but your inability to relax your neck enough to lie at rest indicates tension in the whole core of your body.

This situation is symptomatic of a perpetual leaning forward, which indicates that some tension exists in the muscles on the front of the neck where it joins the shoulder girdle at the chest above the clavicle. That tension draws the neck forward and up and demands a corresponding tension on the back of the neck to act as a counterbalance. But the compensatory tension literally makes the neck too short to lie down flat at rest. One of the first tasks of this session, then, is to lengthen the back of the neck and allow it to relax and achieve a greater degree of vertical alignment.

The neck is designed to be a vertical pillar that supports the ball-like head resting on top of it. But usually this vertical pillar leans like the Tower of Pisa, so that the ball is inclined to roll off it in a forward direction. Under these circumstances the head requires tension in those muscles in the back of the neck in order to keep from rolling off its tilted pillar. If you feel behind your head right now, behind your ears, and continue to move your fingers forward, you will discover a fascial connection linking the muscles of the back of the head to structures in the face. This connection is something like a band of muscle that attaches to the skull behind the ears and reaches across the joint of the jaw and the eyes, as well as the forehead and temples. This band is probably tight, even as you touch it.

At twelve to fifteen pounds, the average adult head is a considerable weight. When it does not rest easily on top of the neck it becomes a burden the rest of the body has to work to bear. The first vertebra is called the atlas, after the Titan whose chore was to support the heavens on his shoulders. Most people do indeed carry the weight of their whole worlds there at the base of the neck.

Sit squarely with your back straight and well into your chair rather than leaning in any direction, and place your neck in as vertical a position as you comfortably can. Don't push your neck or strain it, simply bring it back over your shoulders. Now gently turn your head, slowly at first, to the left and then to the right. Ideally, you will feel something like concentric cylinders revolving around each other inside your neck, but more likely you will feel a center column around which muscles seem to wrap and unwrap. This feeling is one early indication of tension in your neck.

Next, let your neck lean forward; then raise your head and look straight ahead. Now turn your head left and right. You can see immediately how greatly the position of your neck impairs its free turning. However much or little tension you felt in the first position, it is scant compared with the tension you feel when you stick your neck out.

THE FACE

The face is both the most conspicuous part of the head and that part of the body to which we are most attached emotionally, as the representative and expression of our principal identity. Not only do we put our faces on our driver's licenses, passports, and other identification papers, but we pay a great deal of attention to how our faces look to ourselves and to other people.

Ideally, the face at rest—asleep, for instance, or in a meditative trance—is impassive. As thoughts and feelings arise from our bodies they find expression in our faces; and when they are completed they pass and our faces can return to their rest, or neutral, state.

The Japanese traditionally encourage much more severely than we do the idea of maintaining an immobile and impassive face, no matter what joys or tragedies a person might be facing. The object is to prevent the person facing you from reading anything at all in your face. While the blank slate provides an intriguing mirror on which another person may read or project his own expressions, a more important social feature is that it prevents you from losing face. The blank slate so imposed demands fully as much effort to uphold as any other false expression, of course.

205

There will be time, there will be time
To prepare a face to meet the faces
that you meet. . . .
—T. S. Eliot,
The Lovesong of J. Alfred Prufrock

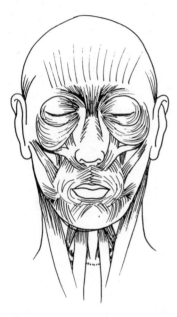

Figure 12-3. Musculature of the face, front view.

People sometimes discover the effort required to maintain a mask when they laugh so hard the muscles in their faces ache. Put a fixed smile on your face now, and hold it frozen for a full minute. The release you experience when you let the smile go is the same sort of release that occurs when you let go of unconscious tension patterns of holding in your face.

But face it: In common practice, most people want to put on a good face, and they carry their favorite expressions on their faces most of their waking lives. Some people have one habitual expression, others have two or three. One person may always look bemused; another may be bug-eyed under one set of circumstances and scared-looking under another. Among the most common habitual expressions in our culture is the plastered-on smile, whose purpose is generally to deceive others into thinking the smiler feels terrific and everything in his life is great. But whether we smile, frown, sneer, or plead, look pleased, stern, or beguiling, a great deal of body tension is required to maintain any false face.

Persona means "mask" in Greek. When actors donned masks to perform theatrical roles in ancient Greece they literally put on different *personae*. In psychology we still consider these personae—the faces we present to the world—in our personalities, and in anatomy we refer to the superficial musculature on the front of the skull, which activates our facial expressions, as the facial mask. From that point of view as well as from the vantage of structural integration, a fixed expression on the face can be maintained only by tension or holding in the muscles.

It is not always true, but quite often people who learn to recognize their masks will find that the expressions they use for holding—their habitual presentations—cover up the expression of other emotions they may have wished to hide from other people or even from themselves. The plastic smile may cover up deep sadness or anger, for example, and the release of the tension that holds the false smile in place may be followed by the release of emotions held captive underneath. Increasing the fluidity of the emotions stimulates the fluidity of emotional expression.

Any mask demands effort and tension to maintain,

and so diminishes the flowing life of the person who must maintain it. A mask is static, an expression of deadness, not of life. The liberation of the face along with the liberation of the emotions that lie behind the mask quite literally mean the liberation of vitality and freedom from deadness.

We said earlier in this book that psychological health is indicated in part by a person's ability to move freely from one feeling to another without being bound by convention, beliefs, or the feelings of moments past. The same is true with regard to *expressing* those feelings, and the face is one of our principal means of emotional expression. When a rigid mask is your whole presentation you cannot be self-expressive, just as when you are fully self-expressive all the aspects of who and how you are become available for self-fulfillment and relationship. And you return flexibility to your whole body and being as you return it to your facial mask.

Part of the work in the seventh Hellerwork session is to allow the client to let go of her habitual expression so that her face may return to neutrality—being at rest when she has nothing going on, and available for expression when she has something to express.

SAVING FACE

People are often amazed to discover that there are muscles beneath the skin of their faces and that they store tension there. The face is the location of most sense organs, which receive and communicate information from and to the world beyond our individual skins. When people learn to experience their patterns of facial holding and let go of these patterns, they can express themselves more clearly and powerfully, and they can feel in a way they never have before. For instance, some Hellerwork clients find they can smell and breathe better when their

Bill: When I was learning to meditate, my face would fall through a series of postures reaching from the expression I was wearing—literally wearing, like a mask or like clothes—to a neutral state. I thought about it then in terms of different valences, personae, and even lifetimes; but another way to understand the progression is that I moved through a set of tensions each time I began a meditation. Early in my studies I would spend some minutes studying the masks as I moved through them, and eventually I became able to move through them very rapidly. Of course, by then there were fewer masks to move through, too. But whether there were many masks or configurations of tension that stood between my self and my self-presentations, or just a few, it was the state of neutrality, when my face was no longer doing its dance, that told me I had reached the point at which meditation itself had become possible.

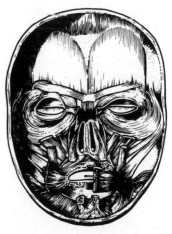

Figure 12-4. Musculature of the facial mask.

207

Bill: I remember how different my voice sounded after this session—much fuller and rounder, as if it was coming from the bottom of a well deep inside myself—and how different my mask looked on videotape from the way it had looked before we began the session. It actually became far more symmetrical. Where one eye had been higher than the other, both eyes looked back at me from approximately the same plane. My jawline evened out, and the two sides of my face became equal in length. What was particularly surprising about these changes was that I had not been aware of the degree to which my face had fallen out of symmetry over the first thirty-seven years of my life, even though for nearly two decades I had made a practice of looking at photographs of other people by covering first one side and then the other of their faces, usually seeing two entirely different expressions in a single picture as a result. I had recognized that in the two expressions I was seeing complementary facets of virtually every person—the explicit presentation and the hidden one, the masculine and the feminine parts, the Apollonian reason and the Dionysian passion—and I found it exhilarating and liberating to see the same features merged and balanced in myself. Furthermore, my life since that time has generally become more integrated, which suggests to me that this work on my physical presentation had a transforming effect on my deep psychological self as well.

Joseph: When I was seven years old I fell into a swimming pool at a summer camp and literally drowned. I didn't know how to swim, and I started swallowing water like crazy and sinking and I did that all the way down until I hit bottom. Then, all at

nasal passages are released. They become bright-eyed, see better, and laugh and cry more freely when the muscles of their eye sockets are opened. TMJ disorders may clear up, and teeth grinding may stop when jaws and mouths are realigned. People hear better and lose a sense of ringing in the ears when their auditory passages are clear and not constricted. Stammers and stutters sometimes disappear as people become less tongue-tied. And finally, nearly everyone begins to realize how much effort he or she has had to exert to present and maintain some immobile persona that actually belied the fluidity of what was taking place inside them all the time. As a result of this freedom, of course, people generally experience enormous relief.

Tension in the head, neck, face, jaw, and mouth affects our voice tones measurably. Such changes are easily recognized when, as a result of easing tension in the vocal cords, the voice becomes more efficient and capable of a greater tonal range, and when the lessened tension throughout the head allows the skull to act as a resonating chamber, with sounds amplified in all the cranial cavities just as they are in the sound box of a violin or guitar. Indeed, singers are trained to project their voices through the facial mask in such a way that the voice does rise and resonate in the head, in order to achieve the famous round, pear-shaped tones instead of thin, reedy ones.

One result of the work on the face is that people tend to look younger. The appearance of what we call "aging" is often the result of fatigue, strain, and tension in the face, expressed in wrinkles, sagging musculature, and skin that has either too much or too little face to cover. When these symptoms go away, which is one result of integrating the head, the face shows less wear and tear, and people *do* look younger. People also look younger after the head session because their eyes shine with a sense of vibrancy, energy, and connection to their cores.

Tension in the neck usually involves tension in the lower jaw and inside of the mouth as well, because although most people think the neck stops at the floor of the mouth, the whole lower jaw actually hangs suspended from the skull in front of the neck, stopping at approximately the level of the upper lip. In most integrative bodywork, important changes in the head are effected through the mouth.

The mouth is one of the first organs through which we learn about the world as infants; it is the entryway to the body for nourishment and the palpable channel for communication. Moreover, as babies we put everything into our mouths as a way to explore the world and discover our distinct identities in it. The mouth quickly becomes a primary area of recognition and expression. Over the years, most of us have repressed innumerable expressions of the emotions we feel, and in the process of restraining ourselves we have tightened our jaws. By clamping them down and shutting them up repeatedly and usually unconsciously, we have made the jaws and mouth very tense. Bodywork in the mouth usually touches this ancient tension deeply, giving rise to many of our buried emotions and to their corresponding responses.

once, the fighting left me and the last thing I remember consciously is lying on the bottom of the pool looking up at the sun through the water. Around the pool were these tall cypress trees which from the refraction of the water seemed to be like long, dark fingers bending toward the sun. My last conscious memory is of going out toward that bright light.

When I was pulled out of the pool I had to be revived, and I didn't want to go near the water again until I was about sixteen. I never even wanted to think about the incident. When I was being Rolfed the work on my mouth brought up all my memories of drowning and swallowing water, and I felt a lot of fear and panic. Afterwards I felt free of these emotions, and also free from other constrictions in my throat.

Cranial Osteopathy

When the features of the head and face have been realigned, we move on to release tensions in the cranial cavity itself. As one way of understanding this piece of work, let us digress for a brief exposition of an unusual bodywork specialty called cranial osteopathy.

Cranial osteopathy is the study and treatment of the articulation of bones in the cranium, developed by William Sutherland at the turn of the last century. According to common medical theory, these bones are joined and articulated through their sutures, which become fused by about the age of thirty, effectively turning the cranium into a single piece of bone. According to Sutherland, however, the sutures remain articulated throughout life. The different sections of the cranium move at these seams, their constant expansion and contraction acting as a pumping mechanism to move cerebrospinal

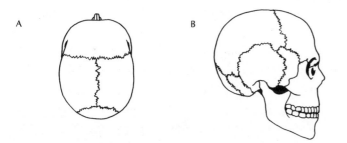

Figure 12-5. Skull with sutures (A: top view; B: side view).

fluid up and down the spinal cord and around the brain.

The brain and spinal cord are contained in a membrane of connective tissue called the *dura mater,* which means "hard mother." This membrane, which laps the entire brain and continues down the spinal cord into the sacrum, is filled with the liquid connective tissue cerebrospinal fluid. The fluid constitutes a kind of hydraulic suspension for the central nervous system, absorbing shocks while providing nourishment for the central nervous system. It needs to circulate, and is pumped around the body through the process of breathing and by the movements of the sacrum.

According to cranial osteopaths, the entire dura mater and cranium also pulsate at a slow rate, and it is this pulsation, which they call the primary respiratory mechanism, that precedes and triggers normal, unconscious breathing. By this theory, the lungs themselves breathe in response to the primary respiratory mechanism. Cranial osteopaths work to even out the cranial envelope, enabling the pulsation to occur with the least possible hindrance and leading to healthy breathing all over the body.

Whether the theory behind cranial osteopathy is true or not, the release of tension in the cranium clearly results in the release of tension throughout the body core. Some clients in Hellerwork even feel their pelvic structures released as a consequence, and there is no doubt that the cranium at the top and the pelvis at the bottom of the core are intimately and structurally connected if for no other reason than, as Ida Rolf used to observe, the floor of the mouth and the floor of the pelvis are the two ends of the digestive tube.

WHAT YOU FIND WHEN YOU LOSE YOUR HEAD

When you lose your head you have the opportunity to rediscover the rest of your body. In particular you are returned to, or have returned to you, the core issues we have been discussing in the past four chapters. You start to experience the polarity of the head and pelvis as complementary rather than antagonistic, as balance rather than opposition.

Each of us individually reflects the attributes of our society as society reflects ours. This world view does not suggest a causal relationship between ourselves and our world, but does imply that we can see the tensions of our world reflected in our bodies, as we can see our own tensions in the larger body politic. By extension, what we learn about our bodies we can apply to the world around us, as we can apply to ourselves what we learn of that world.

One common result of the seventh Hellerwork session is that the client's head and face become more symmetrical. Ordinarily, cranial symmetry in adult human beings is the exception, not the rule. One side of the face is usually shorter and tighter than the other. Also, one side is usually seen as relaxed, open, and outgoing, while the other appears more drawn, closed, and sinister. In effect, the asymmetry reflects two predominant sides of a personality. The session on the head is intended to increase the balance and integration between these two sides, not only of the physical head and face, but of the mental and spiritual faces as well.

Ultimately, losing your head involves achieving a balance of reason and passion, and that is the goal we aim for when straightening all of the body core. The work of structural integration is physical, but it necessarily involves the mind and spirit, since balancing the body entails balancing its energies. The throat, forehead, and crown of the head are the traditional seats of the three upper energy centers, and when they are vertically aligned they allow energy to flow through the metaphysical structure as the vertically aligned body allows energy to flow through the physical one. Whether you choose to look at the body in anatomical or spiritual terms—rationally or passionately, as it were—alignment means the nerves and channels are not impeded: The flow of blood, the flow of cerebrospinal fluid, and the flow of psychic energy are not clamped off, and everything can pass freely through the channels of the body.

Your reason and your passion are the rudder and the sails of your seafaring soul.

If either your sails or your rudder be broken, you can but toss and drift, or else be held at a standstill in midseas.

For reason, ruling alone, is a force confining; and passion, unattended, is a flame that burns to its own destruction.

Therefore let your soul exalt your reason to the height of passion, that it may sing;

And let it direct your passion with reason, that your passion may live through its own daily resurrection, and like the phoenix rise above its own ashes.

... Among the hills, when you sit in the cool shade of the white poplars, sharing the peace and serenity of distant fields and meadows—then let your heart say in silence, "God rests in reason."

And when the storm comes, and the mighty wind shakes the forest, and thunder and lightning proclaim the majesty of the sky—then let your heart say in awe, "God moves in passion."

And since you are a breath in God's sphere, and a leaf in God's forest, you too should rest in reason and move in passion.

—Kahlil Gibran, *The Prophet*

THE BALANCING ACT

13

MASCULINE AND FEMININE ENERGIES

The eleven Hellerwork sessions recapitulate identifiable stages in the process of growing up. The first three sessions, reflected in the chapters "Inspiration," "Understanding," and "Reaching Out," concern issues of infancy and early childhood: breathing, independence, and aggression. The core sessions—"Control and Surrender," "Gut Feelings," "Holding Back," and "Losing Your Head"—deal with issues that come to the fore in adolescence: puberty, controlled surrender, self-expression, and merging the capacities for thought and feeling.

With the last four sessions, which constitute the last two chapters of this book, we sum up all that has come before in the central issues of adulthood: finding our balanced, autonomous identity and integrating it into our lives. The process we are engaged in, then, is considerably more than simple physical manipulation: As the body is the hologram of the being, so Hellerwork is a process of *realizing* that being in the flesh.

Balancing complementary energies is essential to the psychological process of becoming fully mature, and when a misaligned body becomes balanced, there is often a corresponding growing up—a measurable lengthening of the body. These processes are concluded in the two Hellerwork sessions that parallel this chapter.

ON BALANCE

When you were a child you may have tried to stand at the fulcrum of a teeter-totter or seesaw. Your arms would have been thrust out to your sides, and they, like you and like the seesaw itself, would have wavered up and down like the balance plates on a delicate scale. In your small way you would have resembled a tightrope walker, finding stability in movement on your inherently unstable perch.

You can simulate those feelings of balance/imbalance now by standing on one foot while you peel an orange, or tie the shoe on the foot of your raised leg. You will experience some constant rocking back and forth from front to back, and from the inside to the outside of your foot. To some degree you will busy yourself with not falling, and you may forget something about your manual activity, or do it less well than you would under more stable conditions. In any case a certain amount of your attention will be diverted to the process of keeping your balance, and the less stable you are standing on one foot, the more your attention will have to be devoted to that process. Nearly every tightrope walker carries a pole or umbrella or other balance object, but very few juggle while they walk the wire, and we in the audience intuitively appreciate the added difficulty for those who do.

In bodywork we are concerned with numerous manifestations of balance: left and right, up and down, front and back, inside and outside. It can even be said that balance is at the heart of bodywork, and that all the attention we pay to particular parts along the way is primarily a means of balancing the body's components so that we can return the whole structure to balance on the strength of balance, rather than trying to balance a set of imbalances, which is essentially the process that led each of us to an imbalanced state in the first place.

Although we seek balance in every pair of the body's complements, the balance between the upper and lower halves of the body demands our special consideration, for here we can see most readily the interplay of the two dominant embodied principles of life: feminine and masculine energies. Both physically and metaphysically, the lower part acts as our feminine aspect, providing us with support and grounding. Through our feet and legs we stand firm in our direct contact with Mother Earth; our abdomens draw our attention inward to the mysteries of passion, intuition, and receptivity. Similarly, our upper parts act as our masculine aspects. Through the upper part of our bodies we reach out to the world around us with our arms, and use our heads to order our explorations and communications with reason, thought, and penetration.

Not only the upper and lower parts of the body but

also the core and sleeve muscles must be balanced; otherwise, the body cannot rotate smoothly about its vertical axis. Almost everyone is turned in one direction or another to some slight degree, but the amount of rotation itself is rarely significant, and most people never even become aware of it. If you do have a rotation, it can be seen in the commonest sorts of everyday activity, such as generally turning to the left or the right when circumstances do not dictate either direction. Note which way you cock your head when talking with another person, or which way you turn your face when you go to sleep at night.

If you take a walk back and forth across the room you are in right now, which way do you want to turn when you approach the wall? If you ski, or skate, or swim laps, do you sometimes feel there is only one way to turn? Earlier in this book we asked you to fold your arms and then to fold them again the other way, and we observed that the second way probably felt vaguely "wrong," even though there is no anatomical reason it should feel that way. In your feelings about which way is "right" for you, you can discover the direction of your own habitual rotation.

In simple terms, your pattern of rotation *is* just habit. Moshe Feldenkrais called it a neuromuscular pattern, and as he has observed, such a pattern will continue unless something comes along to perturb it. There is nothing inherently bad about such habits. What *is* problematic, though, is that when you remain unaware of them, things may sometimes appear to be happening *to* you, out of your control, which you *could* have an effect on if you wished. It is no surprise, for example, that some accident-prone people keep banging their right hips, right hands, and right legs (or their left; the point is the consistency of the pattern): Their bodies are chronically turned the slight degree that keeps their right sides protruding enough to be in the way of their otherwise balanced acts. By moving toward rotational or any other balance, we move toward freedom.

There is very little in our upbringing that teaches us the basic facts of balance, and we have so constructed our lives that they constantly reinforce our experience of imbalance. At different times in this book we have talked about the unnatural act of walking in shoes with heels on hard, flat surfaces; we have talked about the imposition of reason on passion and the valuation of the extrinsic muscles over the intrinsic ones; we have talked about requiring children, as well as adults, to sit still for hours at a time during the day; and we have talked about the general rigidity of our architecture and furnishings, most of whose formal lines and angles can be found in nature only as aberrations. All in all, we seem determined to impose human consciousness on our environment, aiming to conquer rather than to live in harmony with nature.

But balance is harmony, not precision. Every apple ripens on its own schedule: the tree does not expect all its apples to come ripe on the same day at the same hour. We do want the railroads and airlines to keep to timetables, but when we try to make everything else in life run on a similarly precise schedule, we are asking the head to be disengaged from the body, the mechanical to be imposed on the living, the masculine energy to be imposed on the feminine. Part of what becomes apparent when we examine the body from a biofunctional perspective like that of Hellerwork is that, whether they teach us or reflect us, all these imbalanced approaches to living are intimate expressions of chronic imbalance *in our bodies*.

Balance takes place only in relationship: You can only be balanced relative to something. Being centered is being balanced, and being off-balance is being off-center. The process of becoming balanced, in Hellerwork as elsewhere, is the process of finding your center.

Joseph: In my training program I have people work strenuously and intensively for an hour or so, and then we have a break where everyone gets up to dance for a few minutes; sometimes we lie on the floor and listen to music. Both the movement of the body and the movement in the focus of our attention are refreshing, and they allow us to return to work with more energy and higher spirits. Ultimately, we accomplish more and accomplish it better than we would just grinding through the course. But even more important is that the work becomes satisfying, and job satisfaction is the second component, along with results, that makes for successful work.

In looking at the relationship—the balance—between the upper and lower halves of the body once more, we see that the activity expressed by the former depends upon the stability of the latter for support as a platform from which action can arise. Ultimately, that platform is the ground we stand on. When that ground becomes unstable we have the experience of the bottom dropping out, which leaves us no place to stand.

Archimedes said he could move the world if he but had a place to stand. Of course the corollary is that without a place to stand it is effectively impossible to move anything. In a small way you might have had such an experience playing with an inflated ball in water that was deep enough to keep you from reaching bottom. When you tried to throw the ball you sank somewhat, because water provides almost no grounding, no resistance under your feet.

MASCULINE/FEMININE

Physical imbalances are reflected in the body's proportions. For example, someone who plays a great deal of tennis is likely to have developed one arm and one side of the chest more highly than the other arm and other side of the chest. One imbalance commonly seen in the modern Western world is the woman whose heavy hips and thighs support a thin upper body; another is the thin-legged, barrel-chested man. She is so heavily grounded in her feminine energy that she holds it down and feels less able to fulfill herself in the world than she might. Basically ungrounded, he may do a great deal but is liable to feel insecure and unstable about his accomplishments.

Light and dark, bitter and sweet, more and less—imbalance, like balance, concerns the whole concept of opposites. But where balance is about harmony, imbalance is about choosing one side over the other. When the relationship between elements is not antagonistic, it can be complementary—one of friendly support.

At one level we are involved in a culturewide conspiracy to choose a specific kind of imbalance. For many of us, our choices have become fixed. For example, the barrel-chested man with spindly legs has, in a sense, chosen to look potent in masculine, top-of-the-body activities at the expense of building support and grounding for himself. His choice may have been quite appropriate when he made it. If he was a child dealing with an upper-body issue such as shooting baskets, he may have needed such a focus. And if he devoted himself heart, mind, and free time to his upper-body activity for a day, a week, or even a year, and then he integrated what he had learned into the rest of his life, he would not necessarily have developed his imbalance. But if he made the original choice and forgot about it, he perpetuated the development of his upper body to the exclusion of his lower body. He got stuck in this mode of behavior and his body developed in response, as if he had nothing to do with it —which is almost certainly the way it seems to him now.

People generally think of masculine and feminine as if they are virtually the same as male and female, but even though there is an obvious relationship between gender and the quality of a person's energy, they are by no means identical. Everything masculine contains something feminine, and everything feminine contains something masculine. Each of us constantly balances the complementary polarities of these energies in ourselves, with more or less success. It is one object of this book, as it is one object of Hellerwork, to enhance a satisfying balance.

The masculine end of the continuum is traditionally expressed in creativity; its forms include structure, order, purpose, direction, linearity, hardness, rigidity, activity, toughness. The complementary, feminine end of the spectrum is traditionally expressed in receptivity; its forms include flexibility, discovery, yielding to the flow, circularity, depth, passivity, gentleness.

The fundamental experience of femininity has to do with taking in, in a way that is exemplified by, but by no means restricted to, the sexual act. Taking in is not only being penetrated, but also receiving, embracing, encompassing, allowing into oneself, being open to, enfolding: experiences that essentially take from the outside in. The basic experience of masculinity has to do rather with entering, again in a way that is not limited to sex. Entering is not just penetrating, but also implanting, introducing, initiating, putting forward, expressing: experiences that take place essentially in movement from the inside out. These differences may help explain why the masculine so often seems to exclude the feminine, while the feminine generally includes the masculine.

In human activity, we can see the differences between feminine and masculine energy in something as simple as the ways we walk. Walking to the store to buy something you need, like walking to work, is usually expressed through purposive masculine energy; taking a Sunday stroll is more likely to be expressed through relaxed feminine energy. Obviously, both men and women walk to work and stroll in the park; and obviously, there are situations in which one style of walking is more appropriate than the other. The issue, again, is one of balance, not of gender: We seek to be capable of moving both ways fully, and of flowing between them, having both available to us at any time.

In the course of balancing the body, we seek the ability to walk with the ease and relaxation that are appropriate to a Sunday stroll while walking to work or to the store: purposive, but not rigid, movement; maintaining a sense of direction without losing a sense of flow.

In the modern Western world we see power almost exclusively in masculine terms, which we might define as the ability to do things, or as the ability to produce results in the world. We see power in action, and action as the means to power.

In a sense we have no concept of feminine power, because we place little value on receptivity except as something to be used by action. But this does not mean there is no such thing as feminine power. As the receptive end of the spectrum, feminine power is experienced as attractive: the ability to let results come to you.

Feminine energy is not better than masculine energy,

Joseph: I recently wanted a new camera I saw advertised, and since I am very grounded in masculine power my ordinary mode of behavior would have been to look up a half-dozen photo stores in the phone book, call and ask each one about the features I wanted on the camera, find the best price, and drive to the store and buy the camera. I know from experience that this way produces results. I've done it many times and pride myself on being good at it. In this instance I was unable to follow my normal plan because of a lack of time, and so I forgot about the camera. Three days later I was having lunch with a friend at a restaurant he had chosen. When I came out, there was a camera store in front of me with the camera I wanted on sale. I still had to go to the trouble of walking into the store and writing a check, but I produced the result I wanted—of finding the camera—without lifting a finger. I *attracted* the result.

any more than masculine energy is better than feminine energy. A preponderance of either one leads to imbalance. But our Western tradition has generally ignored or denigrated the feminine altogether. We have insisted on *bringing* things to us, rather than letting them *come* to us. Having only half our energy available to us, we have all been impoverished. After centuries of action-oriented imbalance, recent attention to the power of receptivity is at least a moderating force. Both energies are always available. When we use them both, we have the opportunity of balance they afford.

In terms of the body, women rarely do much with their arms, nor do men put much attention on their legs. As extensions of the upper and lower extremes of the body core, the legs emerge from the feminine pelvis, whereas the arms appear near the masculine head. Representing a dominance of masculine energy, men have inclined toward interests and occupations that express hard, rigid, linear, directive experience, while women, representing a dominance of feminine energy, have been more vested in interests and occupations that imply soft, flexible, circular, implicit experience. It has been humanity's—and particularly the aggressive/masculine—peculiar mistake to decide that one energy was desirable and the other not, and to associate energies with genders.

Whether by design or coincidence, the world is a fairly comfortable place for arms, but not so comfortable for legs. Comfort, where the legs are concerned, is generally a matter of disuse: While legs place you in an elevator or on an escalator, sit you in a chair, put you into a car, and otherwise move you to where you can get off them, they are mostly left alone, a more or less forgotten part of the body.

In some "primitive" societies people sit on their legs.

Throughout history, the more upper class you were, the less you had to use your legs. You could ride a horse while other people walked; if you were very rich, people on foot would carry your sedan chair around. Our whole history has chronicled a coordinated effort to retire the legs. This has represented a choice for the masculine: The more we have retired our legs the more we have created a world for our hands. Our remote-control devices are almost universally hand-operated. Foot controls are always secondary, as on cars or pianos. Choosing the head over the pelvis, mind over matter, masculine over feminine, we have created a chronic imbalance in the ways we use our bodies.

In bodywork we find that people are generally far less conscious of their legs than of their arms, as they are less conscious of their core structures than their sleeves. One of the difficulties we have in getting men to experience their feminine sides is that they tend to hang on to their rigid body armor and the masks we talked about in the previous chapter, "Losing Your Head," and not permit themselves to be flexible, soft, and loose.

But since balancing masculine and feminine energies, like balancing anything else, is a constant dance, you can actually watch it take place simply by becoming aware of the incoming and outgoing energy flow.

A PICTURE OF BALANCE

We mentioned at the beginning of this chapter that balance is at the heart of bodywork, and that one reason we balance the body's components is so that we can base our balance of the whole physical structure on the strength of its balanced parts, rather than on the inherent weaknesses of a set of imbalances. From the standpoint of those factors, what does a balanced body look like?

Loose is a word with many negative connotations in a masculine world: loose woman, loose bowels, having a screw loose. Where the word has positive connotations—loosen up, get loose, loosen your tie—it has to do with attributes of feminine energy generally ascribed to particular subcultures alleged to have a propensity for passion, or to vacations from the masculine, "real" world. Our social patterns become fixed and rigid in the same way our bodies do, as if with a kind of psychic collagen, and these patterns are as self-reinforcing as are patterns in the body: Rigidity promotes rigidity, just as flow promotes flow. We are not speaking only metaphorically, but also in terms of the body's functions: Where there is free-flowing breath and the free movement of fluids, there is not the kind of setting-in of the toxins and sediments that make the body tight.

Joseph: Part of what I like as a body-worker is that I am aware of this dance in my work: I am aware as I work that I am exchanging energy with my client. I communicate through my hands, my words, everything I do; at the same time, I receive messages from my client. The state of balance in bodywork is one of passive activity or active passivity, and as with the martial arts it is possible to perform any activity in such a state of balance, holding both directions open to the flow at once.

Inspiration

Most of the time, most of us concentrate on the intake of breath. Although inhalation is a process of taking in, and therefore appears to partake of feminine energy, it actually works as a masculine process of reaching out for air. To pay equal attention to exhalation is to free held breath and, by allowing the flow, to encourage balanced breathing.

Understanding

In terms of balance, understanding is the ability to see apparently opposing points of view at once, and to see them as complementary rather than as antagonistic. It is also the ability to stand on both feet with equal emphasis: to stand in alignment with gravity, knowing which way is up.

Reaching Out

To be in balance while reaching out is to be able to give and receive, to teach and learn, and to embrace and push away, equally.

Control and Surrender

It is impossible to control forces larger than we are; trying to do so only throws us out of balance. Learning to surrender to the natural flow of life, simultaneously allows us to control ourselves appropriately. Controlling our surrender while surrendering our control is an expression of balance in the realms of the mind and spirit, as well as of the body.

Gut Feelings

With the guts, we are concerned with a balanced awareness of the derms and all they stand for. Mesoderm and ectoderm clearly engage far more of our ordinary attention than endoderm, just as action and thought usually occupy more of our conscious lives than feeling, sensing, or intuiting. Even though in terms of the normal body functions everything is demonstrably in balance, balanced awareness requires that we be open to the feelings in our guts, and that they be loose and relaxed so that energy can flow through them rather than becoming trapped. A lot of well-being simply has to do with taking care of your guts.

Holding Back

Balance in holding back entails not holding back when expression is appropriate, and includes being up-front. Balance includes spontaneity, which is the freedom to move with the flow or energy of the moment.

Losing Your Head

As the seat of reason, the head is something like the organizer or director of our lives. But in order to guide us appropriately it must be able to absorb information from other sources, particularly those identified with the guts and the pelvic floor, at the other end of the body core. Reason can be balanced only by passion.

Structurally, the body is designed to be a balanced channel for a balanced flow of energy. In daily life we all alter our natural channel. Through tension and rigidity, we create other structures that redirect our energies into patterns that may satisfy momentary needs but are ultimately unbalanced and/or unbalancing. All rigidities are structures that perturb the natural flow of energy, and that are reflected in the body's physical, emotional, mental, and movement structures. Every philosophy or system of the body, mind, personality, or spirit has named these structures: subpersonalities, character structure, enneagrams, valences, humors, and so forth.

The task of being human concerns balancing all these elements. If one element in the system falls out of balance and becomes rigid, it can in time draw all the other elements out of balance with it. By the same token, attending to any component and bringing it back into balance can return an entire unbalanced system to order.

In effect, rigidified structures are blocks of stored energy. When the tissues of those structures are released, the energy that has been stored in them is freed. Clients in Hellerwork report having increased energy as their bodies are liberated, and having an increased awareness of that energy as well. They therefore have choice they never had before, concerning the direction in which that energy can move. That choice results from the experience of integration.

INTEGRATION AND COMING OUT | 14

EXCELLENCE WITH EASE

INTEGRATION

Do you remember a time—perhaps you were running, or working, or making love—when you were involved with something in a way that allowed it to flow easily, naturally, and gracefully from your body? When your action seemed to just happen, with little effort on your part? When you felt more energetic and vigorous than usual, and felt less tension in your thoughts and actions than you usually do? That experience, which you can recapture in every facet of your life, is the experience of integration.

Integration is an experience of the whole. *Integrity* means a state of being intact, untouched, unspoiled, complete, whole, entire, unimpaired, or unbroken. The word *integration* derives from the word *integer*, which means unit or whole; integer itself derives from the Latin *tegere*, which is the verb *to touch*. So, although it is a slightly fanciful stretch, we might think of integrity as

225

Many people are inclined to perceive the I and the body as two separate entities. In reality, however, there is no separation between me and my body. I am an embodied consciousness, a subject that is incarnated. All my modes of existence are fundamentally in and through my body. My presence to the world and to people is always a bodily presence, and the others are always bodily present to me. I am neither a disembodied self nor a mechanical organism, but a living unity, a body permeated by self. I live my body as that in, with, and through which I am present to people and things.
—Adrian Van Kamm, "Sex and Existence"

being in touch, which embodies the central concept of integration and allows us to consider the body's integration as a kind of awareness—and vice versa.

This chapter, about integration and empowerment, concerns experiencing relationships in the whole body, rather than experiencing parts isolated from one another. It is also about relationships of all kinds: about how you are not just over there while I am just over here, but how we are interdependent, and how, when we get together, our interaction is about what happens between us rather than just the things each of us is doing. Integration is about unified experience.

REVEALING INTEGRATION

In Hellerwork we talk about integration as putting the parts together to make a whole, but we must also point out that that is not exactly what we're doing. If we were actually putting the parts together it would take a lot more than eleven sessions to accomplish the job. The body is obviously already a whole, but we are often surprised by the ways in which its parts are connected: We work on a knee and the client suddenly feels some release in his shoulder, and that relationship is experienced very concretely. So integration for us is not so much a matter of organizing the parts into a whole as it is of revealing the integrity that is already present in the body. The whole is already there, but in the process of bodywork people begin to feel that integration, and they come to an ongoing and growing experience of themselves as an integrated unit rather than as a collection of parts.

When we lose touch with that connection we cease to experience ourselves as integrated. If you look at the body through a microscope, what you see is a bunch of cells sitting side by side not seeming to have much to do with one another. When you back off a little you see that those cells are part of an organ that is much bigger than the cells. If you back off further you see that the organ is not separate from the cells, but related to them in a whole organized set of activities that constitute the organism. We may even carry this microscopic comparison to its furthest extremes, and see cities as the organisms whose cells are its people, and galaxies as organisms whose cells are its stars.

With the body we may lose the sense of connection between our parts in the same sense that in the larger interplanetary body we have lost our senses of connection. Perhaps we haven't lost it; perhaps we never had it. Part of the experience of being integrated is experiencing yourself as fitting in with your family, community, city, nation, world: You see yourself in relationship, interconnected, and of course you don't have to do anything about that: You already are a part of all those entities. The only question is whether you see yourself as John Doe living in your house, living out your life in isolation, or whether you see yourself as John Doe the doctor, who lives in this red brick house at 252 Main Street, Sandusky, Ohio, next door to Jane Roe the lawyer, and across the street from Leslie Loe the Indian chief. In the latter case you are part of something bigger than yourself: You are interconnected, integrated.

THE EXPERIENCE OF INTEGRATION

When we do not have the experience of being integrated, of being whole, life seems hard in virtually every way: Our desires are not fulfilled, relationships are unsatisfying, and we become exhausted quickly doing very little, like a car running on its battery. At these times we are easily fatigued because we experience ourselves as separate from whatever we try to focus on or engage our-

Joseph: When I began to experience my body as a whole, I felt I was less restricted by the limits of my skin. My skin became a kind of permeable boundary, and I began to feel myself in the midst of my environment. In some ways I began to sense things outside my body that I had not been aware of before. For instance, sitting across from you I had always been aware of seeing you and hearing you as a body over there moving around and doing things; but nowadays, in addition, I experience a more general interaction between us: I feel either comfortable or uncomfortable, I am glad to see you and feel the gladness in all parts of my body, perhaps as warmth; or I am angry at seeing you and become aware that I have some glitch, some holding on, some frustration that weighs on my body and impacts it in some rigid, held way that feels like a perturbance in my whole system. I also feel the physical experience of energy: a nonmaterial connection I might translate as the interaction of your aura and mine, or your gravitational field and mine. The totality of what I feel then prompts me or motivates me to deal with it by expressing it and re-establishing our relationship.

selves with: We are not at one with the natural flow of things. When we *are* integrated, however, we can recognize the experience partly because life seems to require no effort: Everything happens smoothly and we do not feel separate from the world. This is the experience religious and metaphysical teachings refer to as being grounded or centered, being in the moment, being in the here and now, being aware, being in touch—all of which are also terms for physical experiences identical to moving from your body's core. This experience results in excellence with ease.

The body is both the vehicle and the metaphor for integration, as we can see in trying to trace the uncertain process of cause and effect within it. Is your left hip tight because you stand forward on your right foot? Well, yes; but is the tightness in your left hip simultaneously the cause of your standing forward on your right foot? Do both leg problems derive from your hunched shoulders? Or do you hunch your shoulders to maintain your balance because your legs are misaligned? And do all three problems derive from your feeling angry at your mate for needing your attention when you're late for work, or from your feeling guilty about feeling angry, or do you actually feel angry because your body is in pain? All these issues may be related, even causally related, but their relationships are not necessarily linear: Each may equally reflect and provoke any or all of the others.

Integrity is circular, not linear, and if you enter its circle at any point you may see that point as the cause of everything else. But if you entered the circle at any other point you could say *it* was the cause and be no less correct. Any discomfort may certainly result from some other discomfort, which may, itself, be the result of some other discomfort, and so on in an infinite regression of apparent causality. But the same holds true for comforts. In order to correct one imbalance without producing another, it is necessary to integrate the entire system.

In this context, the easiest way to free yourself when things get hard in life is to look to the body and find out where *it* has grown hard. Then you can start to understand both literally and metaphorically what the path is out of the hardness, out of the difficulty.

There are successful therapies of various sorts that aim at the integration of the whole person. Some start from the emotional system, some from the thought process, some from sets of attitudes, some from systems of belief. Some, such as yoga and acupuncture, approach the person through the body: acupuncture by balancing the flow of energies in the body without materially adjusting the physical structure, yoga by integrating the physical structure in a deliberate, meditative manner. One of the unique values of structural bodywork is that its systematic approach encompasses the body directly, holistically, and quickly. In that sense, bodywork may be especially suited to our Western 20th-century temperament: We like to get results fast.

Yet the effects of bodywork do not result simply from presenting yourself for a series of sessions and leaving the consulting room with your body "fixed," like a car you leave with your mechanic. Bodywork is an ongoing integral process of awareness and movement in, through, and about the body. At the end of a course of sessions you can take away from the consulting room a new way of using your body in the circumstances of your own life, aware of that difference, its implications, and its effects. You do not merely have the physical experience that your legs, let us say, feel different when you leave the second session than they did when you came in the door; you are also increasingly able to re-create that experience for yourself when you sit at your desk, drive your car, or take a walk. By the time you reach the point of integrating your bodywork you have been able to replicate the expe-

Everything is the cause of anything.
—Ralph Waldo Emerson

Bill: I was driving home after our eleventh session, and what made me recognize that I was feeling integrated was recognizing that up until that moment I had *not* felt that way. In other words, I recognized the absence of an absence. I saw that in my general experience, or what I took to be normal for myself, my arms were my arms and my legs were my legs and my chest was my chest and so forth. And I realized I had always felt that way because for the first time I didn't. I felt I was a single, unified structure. Abruptly, everything fell into place— or, more accurately, I recognized for the first time that everything *was* in place.

229

Bill: I had most of my sessions with you [Joseph] in a building at a ranch, through whose window I could see a large palomino horse. I used to look at that horse while I walked back and forth to feel the changes in my body after each session, and I would compare the way the horse moved with the way I moved. For example, you would tell me to lift my leg in a particular way so that my ankle stayed loose, and I could see that when the horse walked its ankles stayed loose in that way. I was able to model my way of moving on the horse's way of moving, which helped me to integrate the changes I was learning through my body.

rience in your whole body and even your whole life. This, too, is part of bodywork's integrative function.

In the course of Hellerwork, client and practitioner work back and forth throughout eleven sessions to integrate that new experience in the client's entire body so that by the last session he is fully aware of the shift. In a different way, we are seeking a similar change in awareness for you as you read this book, although because we must convey most of the information through the mind rather than through the body, both the awareness and the results may be less direct.

When we learn to move from our body cores, we learn to move the way animals do naturally. Either we civilized humans never had that talent, which hardly seems likely, or else in the course of growing up we lose the facility that may have been ours at birth, learning a way of life that demands our attention to surfaces and appearances—to the outer, superficial layer of things—and losing at the same time the experience of our inner selves.

But when we regain our ability to move as a whole, integrated unit instead of as a set of more or less dysynchronous parts, movement originates in the core once again and cascades out through our bodies to the world around us. As a result, we move fluidly, gracefully, and easily, with an integrated kind of motion that recalls us to ourselves. When the gymnast Nadja Comeneci scored her perfect 10 in the Olympics a few years back, the whole world cheered: None of us could begin to do what she had done, but we admired the quality of her performance, we were inspired by it, and we *recognized* it because we have all had the same experience, if only for a moment, of being fully integrated.

Think of yourself as a surfer on a surfboard, *not* in the flow of the waves. As you ride even a gentle swell, you look as if you have a tight body. Your jaws and fists are clenched, your thighs ache, your neck is stiff, your shoulders are rigid, you're trying to control your board on top of the water that *will* not behave as you want it to, you're engaged in a constant struggle for control against forces enormously greater than yourself, and even if you do not end up falling off the board, your ride looks and feels exhausting. Surfing is no fun for you, and if you come back to the ocean tomorrow you must have some other reason than pleasure to be doing these awful things to yourself.

But when you *are* in the flow of the waves, everything is easy and right: Your body feels graceful and light and liquid as the sea that rolls beneath you like a cradling hand; the wave grows higher and higher and hurls you on ahead, and you notice everything—the water, other surfers, the shore coming at you, the exhilarating rush. Even if you wipe out, you have had a ride to remember, and you will be eager to hit the surf again as soon as you can, for the sheer joy of it.

Joy is one feature of the experience of integration; it is what motivates all of us to do the things we love. Nobody gets on the ski slopes for the experience of clutching the poles and struggling; nobody skates out onto the ice for the experience of trying desperately not to fall down. We work, we play, we love for the ecstasy of the excellence that comes with ease.

Excellence with ease is what happens consistently in conditions of integrity. One of the problems people often have in achieving this sort of experience is the widely held belief that excellence can only be generated by moving heaven and earth, whereas actually it cannot be generated until you stop trying to move heaven and earth and settle down. Too often we separate the experience of excellence from our experience of life. We allow that Nadja Comeneci can have it, but for us at the office, in our own homes, and in our relationships, life is a struggle.

Joy is the most infallible sign of the presence of God.
—Teilhard de Chardin

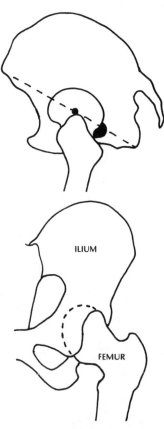

Figure 14-1. Consider a ball-and-socket joint, such as the hip, where the thigh bone (femur) meets the hip (ilium). It is fairly easy to see that this joint is designed to be concentric: The center of the ball and the center of the socket should coincide in order for the joint to function optimally. But when the two centers become different, the joint becomes disintegrated. It is not destroyed, but in being off-center, so that its parts no longer exhibit the relationship they were designed to express, the joint ceases to be integrated and requires more effort to operate.

ILIUM

FEMUR

The challenge that life presents and that integrative body-work addresses is that such excellence and the concomitant experience of joy can be available in everyday life.

INTEGRATION AND THE BODY

In the tenth Hellerwork session we brought the body's joints into balance. The joints are the physical representations of connection; they are relationship. Now, in the course of integration, we bring all the balanced parts together to complete their relationship, looking at the body as a whole rather than considering the knee, for instance, as merely the lower leg leading to the thigh.

When you go to school you are taught, say, science, history, and music as three separate subjects. You learn different things and begin to think of them as having happened separately. You become aware that Galileo, Newton, Pasteur, and Pauling were great scientists at different times in history, and you may become aware that Galileo lived before Newton who lived before Pasteur who lived before Pauling. Likewise in music you may become aware that among the great composers Bach lived before Tchaikowsky and Tchaikowsky lived before Stravinsky. And in the world of English queens you may learn that Elizabeth I lived before Victoria who lived before Elizabeth II. But most Americans with a college education would be hard pressed to say whether Newton was a contemporary of Bach, or whether Victoria was a contemporary of Pasteur. We learned these tidbits of information on different tracks, and we have had little impetus to view them as the whole that history actually is.

Similarly, most of us have learned to see the body as a leg here and an arm there, a chest, hips, aha! another arm, some hands, a foot, another foot *with* another leg, a head, and so forth, and we talk about the body that way: My head hurts; my legs are tired. Most doctors and nurses have learned to see the knee bone connected to the thigh bone, and the thigh bone connected to the hip bone; then, on a different track, they have learned that the trapezius connects the neck to the scapula, and the deltoid follows, connecting the scapula to the arm.

In bodywork we look at everything at once, rather the way you look at a painting: You see the horse, the rider, and the fields—the component parts—but you see them simultaneously, as a single, complex picture, rather than as a series or collection of simple, dissociated images. At the point of integration we see how all the components fit together. We work with the joints to establish the proper relationships so that the body *can* function as a whole, and the client can feel her whole unit moving in concert rather than as a disjointed collection of parts. Ida Rolf used to tell her students that maturity relates to the joints, and upon reflection we can see how that is so. A child starts out with very flexible joints: over-flexible, in a sense, so that there is very little stability. At the other end of the life cycle, the very old person generally has extremely stable joints and minimal flexibility. Maturity is the happy state of balance when the joints are both stable and flexible. Maturity implies the same kinds of qualities we have already described as integration. It suggests the same sense of ease at owning and having a sense of responsibility about your experience, feeling not that things are happening to you or being done to you but that you exercise the kind of control over events that the surfer has over his board when he has surrendered to the wave. Maturity, like integration, entails being flexible enough to create and re-create your own experience, while stability requires that you be adaptable and open to change.

One way maturity seems to come about is through the embodiment of the emotions. Emotional integration

We have bodies, but we are also, in a specific sense, bodies; our embodiment is a necessary requirement of our social identification so that it would be ludicrous to say, "I have arrived and I have brought my body with me."
—Bryan S. Turner

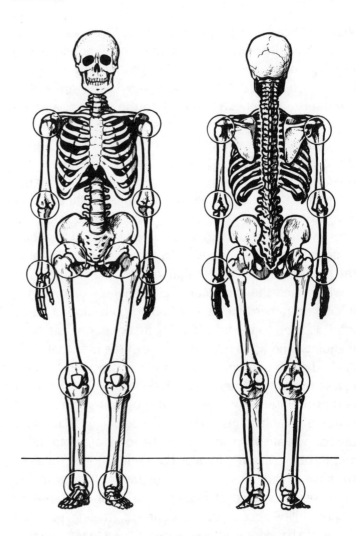

Figure 14-2. The skeletal system with the joints highlighted.

entails a kind of joyful willingness to accept our disparate parts. We all have a part in us that is childish or childlike, through which we become playful, awed, inspired; we all have a parental part that likes to be in control; we all have a vulnerable part that is sensitive and can be hurt; we have a vengeful part that wants to strike back when we feel wronged. Maturity embraces them all.

In the course of growing up we are taught that some of our parts are unacceptable. We're somehow supposed to get rid of these parts, or hold them in. Denying or rejecting facets of ourselves arrests and impedes the experience of integration until those parts of ourselves that we've stuffed down out of sight begin to demand the attention that is rightfully theirs. Eventually they come to dominate our lives.

We see many holding patterns in people's bodies, perhaps because each of us develops somewhat as a plant does: If you do not give a plant the nourishment it needs, it will rarely keel over and die immediately. More often some part of its growth will become arrested and it will grow abnormally. It may not flower, or if it flowers it may not fruit; its leaves may turn yellow rather than green, or pink rather than red.

Similarly, if critical emotional or physical nourishment is not provided to a person at the right time, or if the person cannot incorporate that nourishment, or if it is withdrawn or perceived to be withdrawn when it is needed, the person effectively stops growing in the affected part of herself. Then the stunted part, demanding the nourishment it failed to get, comes to dominate the personality. It also comes to dominate the body. We all know someone who looks like an overgrown baby, and if we think about that person we will arrive at some baby-age she seems to us to be, beneath her social veneer. In fact, we have probably identified an important glitch in the person's emotional growth her body perfectly reflects. As we watch her from our new perspective we will see more and more evidence that her adult life is predicated on some need that was unfulfilled in her childhood, the search for whose fulfillment affects her entire life.

One of the results of integrative bodywork is that people come to look their own ages more uniformly:

Joseph: In my classes I ask the students to look at each other and state the baby ages they see in each other. What amazes me is the consistency of responses: Everyone will agree on the ages for everyone else. When we go around the room and question the members of the class, it nearly always turns out that the age at which he or she has been identified is the age at which some significant, traumatic event occurred: the withdrawal of love or attention or support, for instance.

Another thing that is surprising about this process is that someone can change his own basic age. I had one thirty-year-old woman, for example, who was rather baby-faced and was regularly pegged at three years old. In addition to looking very young, this particular woman had unusually small hands and feet; but over the ensuing weeks she began to look what we call mature. At the same time, in very short order, her wisdom teeth started to come in. And over the next year her hands grew more in proportion to the rest of her body. It may be that part of her manual growth resulted from her activity as a bodyworker, because she was using her hands so that they grew increasingly strong, but somehow that movement was part of the experience for her. A year later she appeared to be a strong, attractive woman.

There ceases to be one part that looks like a little girl and another that looks like an old woman, one part playful and relaxed and another part tight and controlling: People attain increased uniformity in their overall self-presentations. Often that uniformity has the appearance of relative youth, simply because the signs of wear and tear we generally associate with old age have dissipated.

COMING OUT: EMPOWERMENT

As most of us live we feel constrained to give away much of our personal power to people who have been formally trained as experts. Nowhere is this process so clear as in the way we place our powers in the hands of body specialists. But no matter how well trained a doctor, nurse, bodyworker, or physical therapist may be, *you* remain the ultimate authority on your own body. You grew it from one cell without even thinking about it, you live in it—you *are* it—twenty-four hours a day, and you, not the experts, suffer when something is amiss.

At some point we all can recognize that our limitations are self-created rather than externally imposed. Part of the process of maturity is to stop behaving as if the world is doing things to us. Even though it is valuable to know when you *do* need the help of an expert—as a resource, and not a minor deity—it isn't your boss, your parents, your teachers, your society, or anyone else that is causing your problems: it is yourself, and how you take in and embody what life offers. When each of us reaches this point we can start living life as if it were our own, and take responsibility for the limitations that are ours but have not been foisted off on us. However they got there, they're ours now.

One attribute of bodywork is that it aims to return to you the realization that you have always owned the power in your life, even if you have not always been aware of it or ready to act on it. You gain power by integrating your newly aligned physical structures into your own normal movement patterns. In this way the movement of your everyday activities takes on an easy, balanced, graceful flow; you become increasingly open to the process of change that life is, and to your own participation in that process; you adapt yourself to the variable conditions of life more easily. Part of this adaptation entails realizing that some states of tension and stress are not to be avoided, but are merely features of the process like any others, as well as learning to distinguish them from those tensions and stresses that are inappropriate and merely habitual. It becomes possible to recognize habit and stress from an unstressed point of view, and then to let them go. Stress, after all, is a fact of life. We cannot avoid stress altogether, but we can avoid the struggle that internalizes it when we tighten our bodies against it.

Coming out, then, means that you can take your new-found ability away from your bodywork sessions to create excellence with ease in your life. It starts with your simplest movements and expands to include every kind of experience. In time it grows to be reflected in your interactions with other people and even with the events in your life. Because what you discover when your body is aligned and structurally integrated is that you *are already* integrated into the world around you, just as your cells are integrated into your organs, and your organs into your body systems.

You may find, months after your last session, that somehow and without any special effort, life has become more harmonious than it was; you feel more in the flow of life, and things just seem to fall into place—which is the reverse of falling apart. You may have the sense of surrendering rather than collapsing, while from your schedule to the arrangement of your closets your life seems to take on a new order, as an expression of the need to have your whole life aligned, balanced, integrated, and at ease. There is something of enlightenment that comes about through integration. Enlightenment is part of the result of going through the process of bodywork in general and Hellerwork in particular; it is part of the process of becoming integrated. It happens in all senses of the word: Clients report feeling enlightened in the sense of having more clarity, as well as in the sense of feeling lighter in weight; it's as if some light has been shed on the subject that they are, leaving them more conscious and aware. The enlightenment extends to having more equanimity, being more at ease, having more compassion, more understanding, and surrendering to the flow of life. People often see enlightenment as a destination, a condition, a place to get to, but we are talking about the *direction,* the ongoing process that, like integration, is never finished.

Recognizing this makes enlightenment something that can happen right now, rather than something you end up with twenty years from now. It is a process that intimately, absolutely, and necessarily involves the body. The weakness of many paths to enlightenment has been to forget the physical component. But enlightenment is not just intellectual, emotional, or spiritual; it is a full awareness that includes the experience of being embodied.

Even among those disciplines that do include the body, such as Tai Chi, yoga, or dervish dancing, the body is ordinarily directed to do some particular activity. One of the objects of Hellerwork is to bring the experience of enlightenment as process into the nitty-gritty reality of daily living. Enlightenment is not something that only happens when you meditate, chant your mantra, listen to your favorite piece of music, or pray to God: It is something that happens every day, in the way you move,

Perhaps the most common trap surrounding the notion of enlightenment is viewing it as a state divorced from the moment-to-moment experience of life, as though it were some kind of paradisical attainment, which transcends earthly existence. People attempt to "reach it" in the same way they might run after a bus.
—Marco Vassi, *Bodhi is the Body*

relate to others, work, cook supper, brush your teeth. The challenge or purpose of life is to experience it as fully as possible at every moment. Your body is both vehicle and metaphor for your process: When the hologram is integrated with the being, the result is enlightenment.

Notes

Chapter 1

1. Ken Dychtwald, *Bodymind* (New York: Jove, 1978), p. xiii.
2. Stanley Keleman, *Somatic Reality* (Berkeley: Center Press, 1979), p. 11.
3. Ken Wilber, ed., *The Holographic Paradigm and Other Paradoxes* (Boulder, Co., Shambhala, 1982), p. 6.
4. Clara Shaw Schuster and Shirley Smith Ashburn, *The Process of Human Development: A Holistic Approach* (Boston: Little, Brown, 1980), p. 33.
5. Ken Wilber, *No Boundary.* (Boulder, Co., Shambhala, 1979), p. 105.
6. Walpola Rahula, *What the Buddha Taught,* rev. ed. (New York: Grove Press, 1974), p. 34.
7. Robert S. DeRopp, *The Master Game* (New York: Dell Publishing, 1968), p. 189.

Chapter 2

1. Ken Wilber, *No Boundary.* (Boulder, Co., Shambhala, 1979), p. 106.

Chapter 4

1. Don Johnson, *The Protean Body: A Rolfer's View of Human Flexibility* (New York: Harper & Row, 1977), p. 73.

2. Joel Kovel, *A Complete Guide to Therapy: From Psychoanalysis to Behavior Modification* (New York: Pantheon Books, 1976), p. 131.

3. Alexander Lowen, *The Language of the Body* (New York: Collier Books, 1958), pp. 99 and 117.

4. Compare, for example, the energetic traditions delineated in such contemporary expositions as Carlos Casteneda's books about becoming a sorcerer; Jane Roberts's trance-medium channelings for the disembodied spirit she calls Seth; Michael Harner's approach to becoming a shaman; and Amy Wallace and Bill Henkin's explication of becoming a psychic healer. These are just a few among many discussions addressing similar material at varying levels of sophistication. (For citations, see the Bibliography.)

5. Aldous Huxley, *The Perennial Philosophy* (New York: Harper & Row, 1970), p. 21.

6. William James, *The Varieties of Religious Experience* (New York: Mentor Books, 1958), p. 88.

7. Charles W. Leadbeater, *The Chakras* (Wheaton, Ill., Theosophical Publishing House, 1927). Compare contemporary definitions—or interpretations—of this system in books such as Dychtwald's *Bodymind,* Mishlove's *The Roots of Consciousness,* and Wallace and Henkin's *The Psychic Healing Book.* (For citations, see the Bibliography.)

8. F. M. Alexander, *The Resurrection of the Body* (New York: Dell Publishing, 1971). Because Alexander's technique is one of self-help, and not of externally imposed manipulation, it involves the mind in a process of retraining the body. Yet it does not aim to go *beyond* the body to reach the psyche, and so cannot be construed as part of the psychological tradition; nor to channel energy, and so cannot be considered within the energetic tradition; nor to unify body, mind, and spirit, and so cannot be seen as part of the expressly integrative tradition either.

9. Moshe Feldenkrais, *Body and Mature Behavior: A Study of Anxiety, Sex, Gravitation and Learning* (New York: International Universities Press, 1949).

10. Ida Rolf, "Structural Integration," in Dychtwald, *Bodymind,* p. 12.

11. Alexander Lowen, *Bioenergetics* (New York: Penguin Books, 1976), p. 28.

12. Wilhelm Reich, *Character Analysis* (New York: Touch-stone, 1972), p. 285.
13. *Ibid.,* p. 340.
14. *Ibid.,* pp. 341 and 345.
15. *Ibid.,* pp. 384–385.
16. Lowen, *The Language of the Body,* p. 94.
17. For example, Reich states (in *Character Analysis,* p. 457), "The biosystem has a very low tolerance for *sudden increases* of the emotional, i.e., *bioenergetic,* level of functioning," whereas Lowen defines bioenergy (in *Language of the Body,* p. 18) as "one fundamental energy in the human body [which] manifests itself in psychic phenomena or in somatic motion."

    The discussion of bioenergetics in this chapter is in no way intended to slight the work of Dr. John C. Pierrakos, with whom Lowen pioneered bioenergetics, and with whom he founded the Institute of Bioenergetic Analysis. But Pierrakos has published far less than Lowen and he is correspondingly difficult to cite.
18. Lowen, *Bioenergetics,* pp. 203–204.
19. Kovel, *A Complete Guide,* p. 131.
20. Lowen, *The Language of the Body,* p. 86.
21. Ken Dychtwald, *Bodymind* (New York: Jove, 1978), p. 127.

Bibliography

Alexander, F. M. *The Resurrection of the Body.* New York:
Dell Publishing Co., 1971.

Anderson, Walter Truett. *The Upstart Spring: Esalen and the
American Awakening.* Reading, Mass., Addison-Wesley,
1983.

Anthony, Catherine Parker, and Gary A. Thibodeau. *Structure
and Function of the Body.* St. Louis: C. V. Mosby, 1980.

Ayres, A. Jean. *Sensory Integration and Learning Disorders.*
Los Angeles: Western Psychological Services, 1972.

Casteneda, Carlos. *A Separate Reality: Further Conversations
with Don Juan.* New York: Simon & Schuster, 1973.

——. *Journey to Ixtlan: The Lessons of Don Juan.* New
York: Simon & Schuster, 1973.

——. *Tales of Power.* New York: Simon & Schuster, 1974.

Crelin, Edmund S. "Development of the Musculoskeletal System." *Clinical Symposia* 33 (1981):1.

Davenport, Guy. "Lo Splendore della Luce a Bologna," from
Eclogues. San Francisco: North Point Press, 1981.

Davies, Robertson. *The Rebel Angels.* New York: Viking, 1981.

DeRopp, Robert S. *The Master Game.* New York: Dell Publishing, 1968.

Deutsch, Ronald. *The Key to Feminine Response in Marriage.* New York: Random House, 1968.

Dychtwald, Ken. *Bodymind.* New York: Jove, 1978.

Erikson, Erik. *Childhood and Society.* New York: W. W. Norton, 1963.

Feldenkrais, Moshe. *Body and Mature Behavior: A Study of Anxiety, Sex, Gravitation and Learning.* New York: International Universities Press, 1949.

———. *Awareness Through Movement.* New York: Harper & Row, 1977.

———. *The Elusive Obvious.* Cupertino, Ca., Meta Publications, 1981.

Fuller, R. Buckminster. *Ideas and Integrities.* New York: Collier Books, 1969.

———. *Synergetics.* New York: Macmillan, 1975 and 1979 (two volumes).

———. *Critical Path.* New York: St. Martin's Press, 1981.

Gibran, Kahlil. *The Prophet.* New York: Alfred A. Knopf, 1923.

Hampden-Turner, Charles. *Maps of the Mind: Charts and Concepts of the Mind and Its Labyrinths.* New York: Collier Books, 1982.

Hanna, Thomas. *The Body of Life.* New York: Alfred A. Knopf, 1983.

Harner, Michael. *The Way of the Shaman.* New York: Bantam Books, 1982.

Hill, Ann, ed. *A Visual Encyclopedia of Unconventional Medicine.* New York: Crown, 1979.

Hite, Shere. *The Hite Report: A Nationwide Study on Female Sexuality.* New York: Macmillan, 1976.

————. *The Hite Report on Male Sexuality.* New York: Alfred A. Knopf, 1981.

Hunt, Valerie V., et al. *A Study of Structural Integration from Neuromuscular, Energy Field, and Emotional Approaches.* Boulder, Co., Rolf Institute, 1977.

Huxley, Aldous. *The Perennial Philosophy.* New York: Harper & Row, 1970.

The Illustrated Encyclopedia of the Human Body and How It Works. New York: Exeter Books, 1979.

Iyengar, B. K. S. *Light on Yoga.* New York: Schocken Books, 1979.

James, William. *The Varieties of Religious Experience.* New York: Mentor Books, 1958.

Johnson, Don. *The Protean Body.* New York: Harper & Row, 1977.

————. *The Body.* Boston: Beacon, 1983.

Joy, Brugh. *Joy's Way: A Map for the Transformational Journey.* Los Angeles: J. P. Tarcher, 1979.

Kapit, Wynn, and Lawrence M. Elson. *The Anatomy Coloring Book.* New York: Harper & Row, 1977.

Keleman, Stanley. *Somatic Reality.* Berkeley: Center Press, 1979.

Kira, Alexander. *The Bathroom* (rev. ed.). New York: Penguin, 1976.

Kirkby, Ron. "The Probable Reality Behind Structural Integration: How Gravity Supports the Body." Privately printed, n.d.

Korzybski, Alfred. *Science and Sanity: An Introduction to Non-Aristotelian Systems and General Semantics* (4th ed.). Lake Shore, Conn., Institute of General Semantics, 1958.

Kovel, Joel. *A Complete Guide to Therapy: From Psychoanalysis to Behavior Modification.* New York: Pantheon Books, 1976.

Laing, R. D. *Wisdom, Madness & Folly: The Making of a Psychiatrist.* New York: McGraw-Hill, 1985.

Leadbeater, Charles W. *The Chakras.* Wheaton, Ill., Theosophical Publishing House, 1927.

Lockhart, R. D. *Living Anatomy: A Photographic Atlas of Muscles in Action and Surface Contours.* London: Faber and Faber, 1974.

Lowen, Alexander. *The Language of the Body.* New York: Collier Books, 1958.

———. *Bioenergetics.* New York: Penguin Books, 1976.

Memmler, Ruth Lundeen, and Dena Lin Wood. *Structure and Function of the Human Body.* Philadelphia: J. B. Lippincott, 1983.

Miller, Jonathan. *The Body in Question.* New York: Vintage Books, 1982.

Mishlove, Jeffrey. *The Roots of Consciousness: Psychic Liberation through History, Science and Experience.* New York: Random House, 1975.

Moss, Thelma. *The Probability of the Impossible.* Los Angeles: J. P. Tarcher, 1974.

Naisbitt, John. *Megatrends: Ten New Directions Transforming Our Lives.* New York: Warner, 1983.

Perls, Frederick. *Gestalt Therapy Verbatim.* Lafayette, Ca., Real People Press, 1969.

Rahula, Walpola. *What the Buddha Taught* (rev. ed.). New York: Grove Press, 1974.

Reich, Wilhelm. *The Murder of Christ.* Orgonon, Rangely, Maine, Orgone Institute Press, 1953.

————. *Character Analysis.* New York: Touchstone, 1972.

————. *The Function of the Orgasm.* New York: Simon & Schuster, 1973.

Robbie, David L. "Tensional Forces in the Human Body." *Orthopaedic Review* 6 (November 1977):11.

Robbins, Tom. *Even Cowgirls Get the Blues.* New York: Bantam Books, 1977.

Roberts, Jane. *The Nature of Personal Reality: A Seth Book.* Englewood Cliffs, N.J., Prentice-Hall, 1974.

————. *Adventures in Consciousness: An Introduction to Aspect Psychology.* Englewood Cliffs, N.J., Prentice-Hall, 1975.

Rolf, Ida P. *Rolfing: The Integration of Human Structure.* Santa Monica, Ca., Dennis Landman, 1977.

————. "Structural Integration, Gravity: An Unexplored Factor in a More Human Use of Human Beings." Boulder, Co., Rolf Institute, 1962.

————. "Structural Integration: A Contribution to the Understanding of Stress." *Confina Psychiatrica* 16 (1973):69–69.

————. "The Vertical-Experiential Side to Human Potential." Boulder, Co., Rolf Institute, 1977.

————. "Structure: A New Factor in Understanding the Human Condition." Boulder, Co., Rolf Institute, 1978.

Rolf Institute. "The Body Is a Plastic Medium." Boulder, Co., Rolf Institute, n.d.

Schuster, Clara Shaw, and Shirley Smith Ashburn. *The Process of Human Development: A Holistic Approach.* Boston: Little, Brown, 1980.

Sheldon, William. *The Varieties of Temperament: A Psychology of Constitutional Differences.* New York: Harper Bros., 1942.

Silverman, Julian, et al. "Stress, Stimulus Intensity Control, and the Structural Integration Technique." *Confina Psychiatrica* 16 (1973):201–219.

Sweigard, Lulu E. *Human Movement Potential: Its Ideokinetic Facilitation.* New York: Harper & Row, 1974.

Toben, Bob. *Space-Time and Beyond.* New York: E. P. Dutton, 1975.

Todd, Mabel Elsworth. *The Thinking Body.* Brooklyn, N.Y., Dance Horizons, 1972.

Turner, Bryan S. *The Body and Society.* New York: Basil Blackwell, 1985.

Van Kamm, Adrian. "Sex and Existence." In *Readings in Existential Phenomenology,* edited by N. Lawrence and D. O'Conner. Englewood Cliffs, N.J., Prentice-Hall, 1967.

Vassi, Marco. *The Erotic Comedies.* Sag Harbor, N.Y., The Permanent Press, 1981.

von Durkheim, Carlfried Graff. *The Way of Transformation: Daily Life as a Spiritual Exercise.* London: George Allen & Unwin, 1971.

Wallace, Amy, and Bill Henkin. *The Psychic Healing Book.* Berkeley: Wingbow Press, 1981.

Whorf, Benjamin L. *Language, Thought, and Reality.* Out of print.

Wilber, Ken. *No Boundary.* Boulder, Co., Shambhala, 1979.

———. ed. *The Holographic Paradigm and Other Paradoxes.* Boulder, Co., Shambhala, 1982.

INDEX

About the Authors

JOSEPH HELLER, a graduate of Cal Tech, spent ten years as an aerospace engineer at the Jet Propulsion Laboratory in Pasadena, California, where he gained extensive experience of structural stress. He later became the director of Kairos, a Los Angeles center for human development, and participated in year-long training programs in bioenergetics and gestalt, as well as shorter workshops with Buckminster Fuller, John Lilly, Virginia Satir, and Brugh Joy. He became a Rolfer in 1972 and continued to study with Ida Rolf through 1978, while learning Patterning from Judith Aston. He became the first president of the Rolf Institute in 1975 and left that position to found Hellerwork in 1978. He lives, practices, and teaches Hellerwork in Mill Valley, California, and may be reached at 147 Lomita Drive, Suite H, Mill Valley, California 94941; (415) 383-4240.

WILLIAM A. HENKIN holds graduate degrees in both English and psychology. A former university English instructor and magazine editor, he is author or coauthor of fourteen books and editor or producer of a dozen more, including *The Psychic Healing Book* (with Amy Wallace);

Carl Levett's *Crossings: A Transpersonal Approach;* and Karen Preuss's photo-essay, *Life Time: A New Image of Aging.* He has contributed to more than three dozen literary and professional magazines ranging from *Tri-Quarterly* and *New American Review* to the *Journal of Transpersonal Psychology* and the *Journal of Counseling and Development.* A certified Humanist Counselor, AHA, he works in a transitional home for people in mental and emotional crisis. He lives and works in San Francisco.